Naturally Skinny, My Ass!

Healthy Eating Simplified

WRITTEN BY DENICE DUFF

Cover Art and Graphic Design: Erica Falke and Dagmar Torres
Published by: IN YOUR FACE SKINCARE
ISBN: 979-8-9985653-1-1

First Edition
This book is a work of nonfiction based on the author's personal experience.
The information provided is intended for general guidance and entertainment
purposes only and should not be construed as medical advice. Always consult
with a qualified health professional before making changes to your diet or
lifestyle.

For more information, visit: InYourFaceSkincare.com
Printed in the United States of America

DEDICATION

This is dedicated to my Sicilian great-grandmother, who walked every day, cooked like she was still in the old country, and showed me that vibrant health doesn't come from trends—it comes from living simply, moving often, and loving fiercely.

NOTE

Every body is different, and nothing in these chapters is intended to replace medical advice. Always consult your doctor before making changes to your health routine. What's shared here is based on personal experience and what has worked for me.

CONTENTS

Introduction 7

1. La Famiglia..11
2. My First Nutritionist Visit............................14
3. Changing Cities.....................................17
4. "Secret Eating Habits" My Modeling Days..........20
5. My Body's Healthy Bank Account.................25
6. Emotional Eating..................................27
7. The Doomed Diets...............................30
8. The Inconvenience of Convenient Food..........33
9. Your Relationship with Hunger...................38
10. It's Expensive to Eat Healthy... Or is it?..........41
11. The Fat-Free Elephant in the Room..............43
12. Discipline, Willpower, and Other Dirty Words.....46
13. Eat the Rainbow...............................49
14. Peer Pressure.................................52
15. The Restaurant Challenge.......................56
16. Airplanes....................................62
17. Living the Lifestyle...........................64
18. Veggies with Benefits..........................78
19. Onion and Garlic..............................82
20. Tea, My Not-So-Secret Weapon.................85
21. Rethinking Sweetness...........................88
22. My Chinese Neighbors.........................91
23. The Married Life Meals........................93

24. MOVE! 96
25. The Free Facilities of Life.. 100
26. Longevity Foods: Wisdom From a 110-Year-Old.. 105
27. My Grocery List, Broken Down. 107

    Foodie Flashcards. 119
    Snacks 120
    Foods That Support Radiant, Healthy Skin 120
    Foods, Ingredients, and Habits to Avoid for Healthy Skin .. 121
    My Shopping List: 122

Recipe Appendix **127**

Conclusion **180**

Endnotes **181**

Acknowledgements. **182**

About The Author. **183**

INTRODUCTION

Naturally Skinny, My Ass...

That's what my husband kept saying I should title this book. It all started when I was 47 years old at a party having a bite of cake. Someone asked me "How do you stay skinny?"

Before I could answer her, someone else cut in and said "Don't ask Denice—she's just naturally skinny!"

The truth is, although it might look that way, it's not the case. But that girl inadvertently got me to look at all the things I do daily to stay "naturally skinny." And it made me look at what some of the hacks are that keep one's metabolism fast while approaching 40... or 50... or even 70.

When I was 4 years old, I watched *The Fantastic Voyage*, a film where Donald Pleasance, Raquel Welch, and their crew are miniaturized and sent on a submarine journey inside the human body. I was captivated, watching white blood cells and muscle fibers react to these microscopic visitors—it was like a biology lesson brought to life. It gave me a new appreciation for the intricate world inside me and the importance of treating my body with care.

And to be honest, I was fully convinced that Raquel Welch was somewhere inside me... and I had no intention of letting any harm come to her by eating toxic food!

INTRODUCTION

This is not your typical health book. It's a reflection of a lifetime of experiences and relationship with food, where I spill all my secrets on how I manage to live a healthy life and look relatively youthful well into my 50s. With this guide, I intend to break the misconception that people like me are just "naturally skinny," and break the hopeless thought patterns that society instills in our day-to-day ability to control our own health.

Whether you're struggling with yo-yo dieting, seeking more consistent energy, or simply wanting to age gracefully, this book is for you. This isn't a restrictive diet book. It's a roadmap to building a sustainable, enjoyable relationship with food which will last a lifetime.

I've been able to achieve these goals without having to take a ton of supplements every day, live in a gym, or do the very latest expensive biohacking routines. The purpose of this guide is to help you be in control over your own body.

If you are on a special diet, these tips still apply and will help you navigate a sane and forever-way to think and interact with food.

So, I'm not naturally skinny.

People automatically assume that I am slim because "That's the way she was born," or "It runs in her genes." My secret lies in making intentional decisions about what and how I eat, which I've been doing since I was 12 years old when I was told I had hypoglycemia. It was then that I educated myself about the dangers of sugar and foods that turn into sugar quickly.

This is also how I became a "label snob." I read food labels with my mom whenever we went grocery shopping and if sugar was one of the top three ingredients, we wouldn't buy it. If something contained more than 10 ingredients, my mom wasn't a big fan of us buying it either.

I come from a family with five generations of healthy women around the dinner table (granted, one—my daughter—was in a high chair). What I saw at the dinner table were women who ate simple foods from their fridges. That's how my mother raised me, and that's how I raised my kid.

I'm not a doctor or a nutritionist. Though I did become certified as a Nurse assistant and have studied nutrition and wellness since my first visit to a holistic doctor as a young girl. When I was 18 years old I got a scholarship right out of high school for UCLA and majored in Chemistry. I didn't graduate as a chemist but that education along with studying Latin helped me to decipher not only the food labels I was raised to read, but also the complex world of skincare ingredient labels. I'm a wife of 36 years, a mom, an actress, a professional photographer, a director, and the founder of an Inc. 500 skincare company: IN YOUR FACE SKINCARE.

The end game of this book is not about having six-pack abs; it's about being a healthier you. It's about feeling good in your clothes. It's about feeling good in your skin. It's about eating like the old country, not the new country. It's about fewer trips to the doctor. It's about having energy from your 30s and well into your 80s and even 90s. It's about living a long, happy, and fulfilling life, being a healthy mom/grandma or dad/grandpa, and being vibrant partners to our husbands or wives.

We have to look down the road. Which is tough to do because we're thinking of today and maybe tomorrow, but that's usually it. So, I get it. I get the pressure. Just know, you can achieve a better tomorrow by making a few different (and simple) decisions today.

By the end of this book, you'll understand how to eat intuitively and celebrate food. I hope to inspire you to spend less time watching cooking shows and more time messing up your own kitchen—cooking imperfect yet nutrient-filled meals and snacks.

Remember, the true main course is your health, your friends, and the adventures that make life truly fulfilling.

-Denice

CHAPTER ONE

LA FAMIGLIA

My grandparents' kitchen was the holiest place in the house. It was skinny but long. To be precise, it was one and a half grownups wide by six cousins long. And, of course, it's where we all gathered. There was one person cutting garlic, another at the electric meat grinder making sausages, and another taking the freshly caught fillets of breadcrumb-seasoned flounder out of the thin layer of hot olive oil, and placing them on a paper towel-lined newspaper to cool off.

I spent all my summers with my lively, healthy, and very loud Italian grandparents. Our diet was made up of simple food. We grew our produce if possible—and if we couldn't, we bought it as fresh as possible.

My grandparents and I ate pasta every day. They always combined it with some kind of fresh-picked vegetables from their garden. From fresh tomatoes and cucumbers to zucchini and basil, they had taken over the whole backyard of their duplex in Queens, NY. Even the plot of land for the clothesline was covered by their mini farm, with the agreement that the neighbors could reap the delicious rewards.

My great-grandmother, Felicia Provenzano, lived with them too. She came to the United States on a boat from Sicily when she was twenty-two years old with her four-year-old daughter (my grandma). They were greeted by the Statue of Liberty as they entered through Ellis Island, and made their home in New York. Growing up, my Nannie Felicia told me, in her thick Sicilian accent, "When you healthy inside, then you healthy outside." She was my queen. It was never lost on me that I was so fortunate to have my great-grandmother in my life until I was 33 years old.

She fought to carry grocery bags into the house well into her 80s. She cooked, cleaned, and dried the dishes and put them away until she died. You literally had to fight her out of the kitchen to sit down and take a break, all the way up into her 90s. My grandmother, who was chubbier, would always yell at her, "Ma, go sit down! Relax..." But even in my tenth year of life, I knew this woman had a quiet mission inside her. She wanted to live long to get her money's worth out of life.

My Nannie Felicia knew that being sick meant expensive doctors, so she never smoked or drank alcohol. I believe there was the occasional holiday drink, but my family was not big on drinking. Booze was expensive and we didn't have a lot of money. My grandfather bought new fishing poles rather than fine liquors.

They worked hard for their money and they hardly ever went out to dinner. I only ate out with my grandparents at family weddings, anniversaries, or milestone birthday celebrations. To them, the food in restaurants was too greasy, or didn't have enough flavor, or had too much salt, too many ingredients, was overcooked, or not cooked enough. And of course, it was ALWAYS too expensive.

Though, growing up I always loved having fast food at friends' houses. But I also always knew that it was a slight betrayal of my healthy heritage and body's health.

My Nannie Felicia always volunteered to push the baby strollers with her grandchildren, great-grandchildren, and my daughter, who became her great-great-grandchild. At 94, she pushed my daughter in the stroller down Bayview Drive in Long Island. I'll never forget that silently serene, yet loudly magical, moment in my life—the fifth generation.

She lived to be 96 and would still walk a mile a day to the senior citizen center until she was 91. She passed away from hospital pneumonia two days after her second hip surgery – an injury sustained while running down the street to greet someone enthusiastically. In her 96 years, she only spent time in a hospital during that final week.

Her vitality came not from gyms or organized sports, but from the rhythm of daily life: tending to her garden, keeping the house clean, and traversing the city on foot and by public transit, having never gotten a driver's license. While others saw taking the bus or subway as a burden, she discovered what so many overlooked – that the simple act of walking offered rewards no gym membership fee could buy.

CHAPTER TWO

MY FIRST NUTRITIONIST VISIT

When I was 12 years old my mom took me to a nutritionist, Dr. Anita, for a check-up. Yes, I had some acne, and I would get a bit out of breath and lightheaded from running during school PE. But from a blood test along with the symptoms she deduced that I was borderline hypoglycemic. Hypoglycemia is when your blood sugar drops too low—like a car running on empty.

She told me that it could be addressed through my diet and proceeded to teach me about the effects of sugar and how something very "processed" also has the ability to turn into sugar quickly in the body. She explained that when your body doesn't have to do any work, it gets lazy, and, soon after, sick. While eating foods in their more natural state, with the fibers attached, keeps your body's metabolism alive and busy. She said that brown rice was better to eat than white rice because it makes your body work harder due to its higher content of nutrients and fiber. I found out that a real potato was better than a processed box of mashed potatoes because the processed potato was basically just sugary carbs.

To my 12-year-old self she said, "You have to keep your metabolism active. You might have been born with a fast metabolism. But you'll need to keep making good choices as you age to ensure it stays fast." And at 59 years old today, her words have stuck with me through my entire life.

During those visits to my nutritionist there were several things I learned which made sense, were stated in simple terms, and didn't cost an arm or leg to apply to my life:

1. Sugar creates more wrinkles in skin as you age.

2. Incorporate some raw veggies in your diet once a day.

3. Your stomach needs healthy bacteria from probiotics.

4. Home cooked meals are usually lower calorie and healthier than restaurants.

5. It's okay to give your body a break from food (now called intermittent fasting).

6. I can keep my metabolism active through my daily habits.

7. Inconsistent is better than never.

8. You need to be your body's best friend.

I will say, in my 20s and 30s following this inspiration was not always easy. I was on a tight budget from pursuing my career as an actress, while also juggling 2-3 side gigs, from waitressing to being a make-up artist. Yet, even through these financially tough times I could still apply a bit of Dr. Anita's wisdom because:

MY FIRST NUTRITIONIST VISIT

1. I needed to look my best as an actress - healthy skin and a fit body.

2. It was expensive to be sick and cost time away from making money as a self-employed artist in the entertainment industry.

3. I was always able to get cheap fruit and veggies even if only at the 99cent store (not organic but better than chips and cake).

CHAPTER THREE

CHANGING CITIES

Your surroundings and the food resources available to you can greatly influence your eating habits. Though I was born on Long Island, NY, my family moved to Los Angeles in the early '70s, and that's where I was raised—among the rich, the famous, and the thin. The near-perfect 75-degree weather, with no humidity and endless sunshine, turned the city into an outdoor playground. Joggers, rollerbladers, hikers, and surfers filled the streets and beaches.

LA was also miles ahead of the curve when it came to health food trends—sprouted grain bread, wheatgrass shots, and bee pollen smoothies weren't just available, they were normal. Grocery stores had entire aisles dedicated to supplements and organic everything, long before "clean eating" was a catchphrase.

Being in the entertainment industry, I was also surrounded by people hyper-aware of their bodies and health. We weren't just chasing roles—we were chasing that elusive, lit-from-within glow.

Then, in 2017, after our daughter moved out, my husband and I decided to shake things up. We sold our house and moved to Manhattan. At first glance, the weather was harsher and the lifestyle faster, but I quickly saw a similar dedication to wellness. In-between the bagel shops and pizza joints there were juice bars, yoga studios, and organic cafés tucked into every other block.

New Yorkers may walk fast, but they're also quick to invest in themselves—chiropractors, acupuncturists, holistic doctors, and vitamin drip clinics were thriving. Wellness was a status symbol, and the demand for health-focused food was met with ease.

I remember on our trip across country when moving to Manhattan, we stopped at a diner in Oklahoma, and I started to chat with the 24-year-old waitress about healthy eating options. She was seven months pregnant with two other kids. She was fascinated by my "healthy diet soda" concoction I always request: 3/4 club soda, 1/4 coke regular. Thats it. There's no need for fake sugar and also no need for SO MUCH sugar when a splash hits the spot! She said she really wants to eat healthier but as a single mom it's so expensive.

Basically, she was like my mother forty years ago, but this young woman had no education and very little resources to make better choices. She said cooking meals for her family and making their own lunch was more expensive than going to the fast food taco stand.

But when we moved down South to Florida in 2020, things shifted. The climate was steamy, and the pace was slower, but what really surprised me was how different the food culture was. You didn't have to look far to find a drive-thru—it was part of the local rhythm. Health food stores were harder to find, and the vibe wasn't so much "quinoa salad and cold pressed juice" as it was "BBQ ribs and mac n' cheese." Farm stands existed, sure, but you had to know where to look.

It made me realize how much your location shapes your plate. Living in LA or NYC, healthy choices were the default—they were on every corner, in your face, and built into the culture. In smaller towns or more suburban areas, the healthy options take a bit more digging. It's not that people aren't interested in wellness—it's just that the infrastructure isn't always there to support it. When convenience favors drive-thrus over farmers' markets, it takes extra intention to eat in a way that fuels you well.

So, when that friend said to me, "Don't ask Denice—she's just naturally skinny," I had to stop and laugh. Because no, I'm not just "naturally" anything. I've lived in places that made it easier to eat well and stay active.

But I've also lived in places that challenge me to create that lifestyle for myself. The truth is your environment doesn't define your habits—but it does influence them. And the older I get, the more I realize that staying healthy and vibrant isn't just about willpower. It's also about knowing how to outsmart your surroundings, wherever you live.

CHAPTER FOUR

"SECRET EATING HABITS" MY MODELING DAYS...

"Secret eating habits" can wreak havoc on your body. It's not a way to control your eating habits, it's an out of control habit. If you find yourself eating in a secretive manner, foods that you blatantly know aren't healthy, or in amounts you know are excessive, I want you to recognize that the embarrassment you might be feeling is correct. Deep down we all want to do what's best for our bodies. Deep down we all want to respect these complicated, gorgeous vessels called our bodies.

We naturally know that what we are doing isn't for our body's benefit, but we "can't stop ourselves" and are betraying our body instead. So of course we're going to feel bad, withdrawing from others and keeping this eating habit a secret.

I went through my dark eating days when I started as a model at 17. An agent told me, at 5'9" and 123 lbs., that my waist needed to lose two inches. Two inches! Up until then I ate healthy and in moderation. I'd have a few cookies and milk with my grandma or a slice of Entenmann's chocolate cake with my uncle every once in a while. But then, when I was told that my already very skinny body "was not good enough" I became overly paranoid of every calorie I ate. Up until then I had never weighed myself, but after that I got a scale. I started on an unhealthy habit of obsessive eating.

I heard from several models of the binge and purge and my desire to "be perfect" and "exactly what the agents wanted" made me adopt this insane "diet." Gosh, even writing that down now makes me want to go back and hug my younger self and tell me to trust my original eating habits. I only saw pictures of other models at my agency, and I wanted to travel the world. And if my "meal tick- et" to do that was to try and lose inches from my waist, I would do it.

It was 1984 and my agents had me go to a spa which specialized in slimming gadgets. The first week I went they plugged me up to an electro-muscle stimulator machine, concentrating around my abdomen and waist. This ear- ly biohacking exercise device looked like something from some brutal Soviet psychiatric ward documentary from the 60s—and here I was in Beverly hills in the 80s, hooked up to it.

Willingly, I laid there. Electrodes stuck to my stomach area by wires, attached to a metal box filled with dials and numbers. I watched the technician raise the dial to where it was "comfortable yet effective" for me. There was nothing comfortable about these little electric shock pulses cours- ing through my skinny body at 6-second intervals. I'm sure

I agreed on a strength that was way too strong, but re-member, I was not thinking rationally I just was thinking, "I want to travel to Japan as a model and THIS is how it will happen…"

After that treatment they escorted me into a room that looked and sounded more soothing to get a compression mineral salt body wrap. There were bamboo plants and a rattan room divider like you see in the Fiji Islands. I thought, "Ahhhh… this is going to be wonderful." They tightly wrapped my entire naked body in mineral solution soaked ace bandages (not unlike the mummy King Tut). Calming music playing, I tried to relax my mind from the stressful thoughts of "This HAS to work!"

About seven minutes had gone by when I began to have a hard time breathing. I would exhale but then had diffi-culty trying to inhale. My ribs were wrapped so tightly that it was compressing not just my waist, but my lungs. I began to "panic breathe," and once you start that, it's tough to mellow out and adjust. So, after probably no more than eight minutes into this 20 minute procedure, I yelled out through the bamboo room divider in a feeble voice…"Help! Someone…can you help me? I can't breathe…hello?!" The technician came rushing in and quickly started to un-wrap me. I felt like I had failed.

And of course, my waist size did not change. Nor would it have if I had stayed in the full 20 minutes. As I found out years later, I have wide-set ribs and no matter how thin I would get, I could never have a 22 inch waistline.

Japan never happened.

At this time, I was a first year student at UCLA, fitting in modeling castings in between chemistry labs. I had a full scholarship, and felt I should study something "Noble and Worthy" of this free ticket, deciding on engineering and chemistry. To be honest, I didn't feel like I fit in with this very "academic, turquoise, t-shirt-wearing" culture. I wanted to be where they drank cappuccinos and smoked clove cigarettes and wore black turtlenecks.

Now, mind you, I didn't drink coffee nor smoke cigarettes of any kind, but I loved my black clothes, so for my next year of college I applied and got accepted to the NYU Tisch School of the Arts. There, I studied acting, directing and photography. I was so creatively busy that food was literally the last thing on my mind.

My mom couldn't afford the school's meal plan, so I ate a lot of popcorn and apples friends gave me from the school cafeteria. I also always seemed to find open packages of coconut rolled dates from the corner international market that I would, well, help myself to before they threw it away. But months of this pushed me to work again, so I reached out to another modeling agency in Manhattan.

I worked some fashion shows and photoshoot gigs. Then, as the school year was ending, I had the opportunity to... drum roll please...go to Milan! The Modeling Mecca. This time they didn't need my 5'9", 123 lb. frame to be any smaller.

When I arrived at my pensione (shared apartment) I was greeted by a darling model my age from the Midwest named Connie. We became fast friends. We were shoulders to cry on for jobs not booked, and fully supportive friends during the few, but happy, successes. We kept each other safe from the strange men that seemed to be sent to escort us to parties. Luckily, my New York street smarts kept us out of trouble.

My eating habits during those three months in Milan were fairly disciplined—for two reasons. First, I couldn't really afford to indulge in pastries or bowls of cereal, and there weren't fast food restaurants or cheap donut shops on every corner like there are in the U.S. Second, I had stopped purging.

I began to notice that when I purged, my eyes got red, and veins were strained around my face. And then I heard a modeling agent talking on the phone about another model who had left the room, commenting on the damage that her bulimia habit had on her eyes, skin and teeth. That was when I realized the actual physical toll this bad habit takes on your face. Your face! The thing I was most wanting to present in a radiant fashion. That impinged with me.

I realized that binging and purging was the coward's way of eating, and I was better than that. I overcame my eating disorder by looking into the negative health effects. I trusted my body but I was betraying it by binging on food. I felt like a criminal, and my body was the victim. It really reminded me to be my own best friend for the long term, both spiritually and physically.

CHAPTER FIVE

MY BODY'S HEALTHY BANK ACCOUNT

I think of my body's health as a bank account, my Body's Bank Account or **BBA** for short, where every decision you make is either a healthy deposit or an unhealthy withdrawal. Just like with money, the goal is to maintain a positive balance to thrive. Eating nutrient-rich foods, staying hydrated, and engaging in regular physical activity are valuable deposits that build up your "health savings." These actions support your body's systems, boost energy, and improve your overall well-being. The more deposits you make, the more resilient and vibrant your "account" becomes.

I am ALWAYS aware of this concept of making deposits in my body's healthy bank account while also keeping a close check on the withdrawals. I may not always succeed in keeping the healthy deposits abundant or keeping withdrawals to a minimum, but I try to maintain an awareness of it to keep myself on track. Just as two bites of party cake might be a bank account "withdrawal," as is grabbing a few leaves of raw spinach once I'm home from the party a "deposit."

Withdrawals come from overindulging in processed foods, excessive sugar, and unhealthy fats, or neglecting self-care through stress, poor sleep, or inactivity. Just as overspending depletes your finances, too many unhealthy withdrawals can leave you feeling drained, sluggish, and susceptible to illness.

It's simply mathematical. A literal numbers game. Which is why I've always been able to adopt this method. Doing *more* of the good and *less* of the bad. This doesn't mean cutting out indulgences entirely—just like you might budget for a fun splurge, you can enjoy a treat or skip a workout occasionally without guilt. The key is to ensure your overall "account balance" stays in the positive column by focusing on daily habits that nourish and strengthen your body. Small, consistent choices, like swapping sugary drinks for flavored sparkling water or adding more vegetables to your meals, can accumulate over time, just as steady saving grows your financial wealth. Treat your health like your most valuable investment, because it truly is!

Here's how I started to look at how a body functions: Do NOT feel pressured to order food that YOU think will reverse the health trajectory of your body. There are going to be many more times when there are zero healthy options in your future…on a road trip, or vacation, a kid's birthday party, or a business meeting, but at a restaurant that has healthy choices you can take advantage of, that's the time to love your body and put a deposit in your "Body's Healthy Bank Account."

CHAPTER SIX

EMOTIONAL EATING

"I deserve to eat it!" "Once I start, I can't stop."

What do you eat in the quiet moments? What do you eat when you're sad? What do you eat when you are celebrating, or as your reward food? As we all know, food can get very intertwined with our emotions.

At some point in life people have moments when they surrender to their emotions. In their efforts to cope with the situation they tend to engage in emotional eating. We lie to ourselves by calling it comfort food. The honest truth is that comfort food doesn't make you comfortable. The comfort and cozy memories are usually about the people and place—not the food. The notion of comfort led by emotions leads you to eat more food than what **your body really needs.**

Emotional eating is a trap, and changing your mind is the way to escape it. No one is forcing us to eat junk—we do it ourselves. Yes, we are bombarded with so much false information: Endless, entertaining TV commercials, convincing us of the joyful, sexy lifestyle of junk food and alcohol. As an actress, I've worked on these commercials in Hollywood and ironically most of these fit actresses don't ever eat or drink the products they are pitching. They respect their bodies too much to put those toxic trans-fat-filled muffins and sulfite-filled breakfast meats into them. This is brilliant marketing, and these images stay with us. When you're not eating it, you wish you were, but when you are you wish you weren't. Crazy, right?!

There were some stressful years for my mom after the untimely passing of my brother. This was the epitome of emotional eating. She would buy the on-sale box of Entenmann's chocolate donuts because it was only 25 cents! She stopped fitting into her clothes, she didn't want to go out and socialize. She stayed home on days off, eating in front of the TV. She felt more tired, and…ultimately, it didn't bring her son back to life.

She went against all the things she taught ME. And I, unfortunately or fortunately, got to see this dwindling spiral of unhealthy habits play out right in front of me. If I didn't believe that a few mindset shifts could totally affect how, when and why you eat, I saw it and believed it then. Though it saddened me, it also strengthened and inspired me. It inspired me to never eat a whole box of cereal and say "I deserve it!" or open up a bag of chocolate covered almonds and say "Once I start, I cannot stop!" Because I can. No one has a gun to my head saying "Duff, finish the bag or else….!!" Nope. It's purely my choice.

Indulging in these unhealthy and high calorie "comfort foods" seems like we are exercising our freedom. Have you ever asked yourself, the freedom of *what*? A perceived idea of what makes us happy? The irony of it all is that after you eat those junk food meals you usually don't feel happy and energetic. Generally, you feel more like napping. And even deeper is the slow but steady attack on your adrenals and damage to all your bodily functions which you need to give you your youthful glow.

It was 15 years later that my mom got her self-love back and was able to make cleaner decisions and not buy junk food "just because it's saving money." She saw that having to buy new larger clothes to fit into was far more expensive than the $3 she saved buying cheap donuts, and the $200 co-pay at the doctor because too many drive thru meals lowers your immune system making those "seasonal" illnesses easier to catch.

CHAPTER SEVEN

THE DOOMED DIETS

I grew up watching my friends' mothers fall into the trap of celebrity diets. Many were from wealthy families and were sweet and smart, but they still struggled with their weight. Even if the trendy diet worked for a while, I would then see them a year later and they were heavier—and blamed the diet. But these diets were all geared around restrictions and fear, and overly strict discipline…eating a couple of almonds more than your daily allotment would put the fear of total failure in you. The diet became the controlling force.

Life works with two energy flows: Cause and Effect. For these women, and maybe even you reading this, the diet became the boss (Cause) while they, and maybe you, became the victim (Effect). Your will and confidence all revolve around what the diet says.

This is not to discount the cases of people with extreme food allergies. This is for the majority of us who are reasonably healthy but are being marketed to eat supersized quantities of fast fried foods all day, every day.

There are corporations who profit billions by getting you to think, "I've worked hard, and I deserve [insert unhealthy food choice]." So, when you fail, it's the diet's fault, not yours.

I clearly remember a woman who carried a lot of weight—she was about 36 and ate a lot of frozen dinners, totally lacking in nutrition. This woman consistently ate French fries, chips, and frozen packaged meals. One day I was having fresh-cut pineapple, and I offered her a piece, and she said, "No, thank you, I'm on a diet."

That blew my mind. I thought to myself, *You just had a bag of M and M's yesterday, but this nutrient dense bite of pineapple is off limits?!* She didn't like her heavier body and was on her third attempt at a Keto diet that year.

This is a classic example of allowing a diet to rule your self-control and not actually being educated on the importance and magic healing properties of real, homemade, simple foods. I realize almond butter and avocados may contain a lot of fat, but the life-giving nutrition they have compared to a pack of a 100-calorie diet cookies, a frozen packaged enchilada, or a diet soda, is night and day.

I've never thought too much about counting calories. What I count are the alive nutrients in a meal. And no, I don't have a chart of alive nutrients that each food has—it's just the overall estimation based on the values I map out here in this book. Is it a deposit or withdrawal to my BBA? Don't overthink it.

For instance, these days I will do things like schlep a bag with chopped meat, some tomatoes and hot sauce and make a fast and healthy chili stir fry in our office kitchen. Three ingredients. No hidden sugars, trans fats, or preservatives, and I control the sodium. The 10 extra minutes it will take me to make it has ultimately been why I can still fit into my high school jeans at 59 years old. And have, as my husband likes to tell me, "The same glow to your skin as you did the day we got married 36 years ago."

Fortunately, my mother kept me educated about the importance of how real food in small quantities will never let you down.

If you ever find yourself thinking "F### it! I deserve this box of cookies!" Just try and reframe that to be a healthier, pro-YOU war-cry like: "F### him, I'm gonna eat healthy and look hotter than her!" or "F### it! I'm gonna go for a jog so I get energized with more ideas for my business!" "F### this! I'm going to make that green drink and fit back into my favorite jeans!" It's just a flip of a viewpoint.

Making that flip is the key to never having to diet again.

What we deserve is the actualized freedom to eat what our bodies need and want. We deserve to research and discover the correct information about what's in our food, so that every bite we take will actually be a deposit to your BBA and not a withdrawal.

CHAPTER EIGHT

THE INCONVENIENCE OF CONVENIENT FOOD

F ast food isn't convenient - you still have to go some-where to buy it, and then you wind up unnaturally full and super-unsatisfied looking at those discarded wrappers and bags in your car.

"Instant food" usually means quick to burn into sugar. Unless it's from a natural or organic store—where they try to preserve the whole grain—"quick" or "instant" usually means a quicker trip to belly fat, unexplained aches and pains, and definitely faster fatigue, because that food isn't giving your body the energy it really needs. It's pulling energy from you.

So, the moral of the story is: fun packaging = *beware*. Try, on a gradient of course, to buy a few less boxes and bags of those quick, ready meals, knowing they are usually empty calories with little nutritional fiber and vitamins.

We are so "expertly" and so constantly being pitched on the idea of junk food being fun and harmless. If advertisers actually told you that those beautiful nachos were unhealthy for you, you might look at them differently. But they are experts in promoting products—not health.

If you are frequently on the go, or have to order from a restaurant, you have to be aware of the hidden empty calories. Restaurants are creating dishes not with your health in mind, but with their profit in mind. They feed into (literally) all the commercial marketing for fried, cheesy, bread-filled dishes. Even seafood restaurant commercials emphasize the melted buttery sauces of the lobster and crispy fried batter on the shrimp.

Selling you the sexy and sociable joys of eating those food-colored, synthetic, "food" concoctions without any remorse or responsibility for what it does to your system is their job, and they do it damned well. Maybe one day, the triple-stuffed cheesy pizza crust commercial will come with a warning—like drug ads do: "Warning: May cause obesity, high cholesterol, shortness of breath, cellulite, depression, muffin top, acne, high blood pressure, heart attack, etc." Until that day, we have to understand that their job isn't to make and keep us healthy. Their job is to sell their products.

If you wouldn't put Coca Cola into a new born baby's bottle—your 20, 30, 60-year-old, etc., body is the same. It needs all the same nutrition, if not more.

Packaged foods might be our time-saving friend, but they are also our body's enemy. It's the prettiest and most fun-packaged ones that usually do us the least good. Most foods you see advertised on TV are lacking in nutrition. So the next time you see a bright colored item at the store which you saw advertised on TV, know that you should not get it.

If a food or chain can afford a national TV commercial chances are VERY good it is preservative filled, vitamin-less, heavily processed, and filled with hydrogenated oils and synthetic dyes.

The more time, money and graphic designs that are put into marketing a food product usually means the less realness you're getting in that food. The extended moral of the story is: fun packaging + TV commercial = *beware even more.*

Choosing to make a change will free you. You don't have to fear the fast-food crutch anymore—remember, it's just an illusion they've sold to us. I believe that junk food shouldn't be thought of as a guilty pleasure because that gives it too much power and respect. It makes us believe that life without junk food can seem boring, and as though we are sacrificing something.

On the contrary, it won't be a sacrifice. It will only lead to less aches, pains, bumps and bulges! And there will be far more choices than you previously imagined. Eat for health, and that's where the true pleasure comes from. No need to mess around with the "guilty pleasure" myth. Make your future guilty pleasures eating an entire fatty avocado, or two big handfuls of high calorie cashews—those are the guilty pleasures that won't backfire on you.

You won't ever be deprived by eating healthy and understanding that junk-fast-food only feeds you inflammation and tiredness.

Just remember: if it's in a package and meant to last for weeks on a shelf, chances are there's little nutrition left in it.

As a (very loose) rule of thumb: *Choose food that rots.*

Having been raised by a single mom on food stamps many times in our life, trust me—throwing away $1.50 of a $3.25 ice cream cone actually still hurts me to this day. But slowly gaining more belly fat and raising my chance of diabetes would hurt me way more!

I'm also the girl who will throw away the leftover cakes and sweets after a party. If it did its job at the party serving up smiles, then voila, its time is done and there is no need to clog my cardiovascular system to just "not waste it." You are not insulting the pastry chef or the bakery owner. But finishing the carrots or the beans or the apple slice…that's more noble and time better spent filling the BBA.

The wonderful thing is, as a grown-up we're the ones that are in control of what we buy, and what we put in our own cupboards. When you think about what kids eat in other parts of the world, funky eggs, weird fish, strange and pungent vegetables. Try and give that to some American kids. Tastes adapt to their environment—generally. The bottom line is, you don't have to buy those foods as an ongoing part of their daily diet.

The best defense for raising healthy children is to educate them early on…and not to get too strict on depriving them of "evil sugar." If your child wants to get something sweet at a market, you can let them know, "I can buy this, but these ingredients will make your body tired, and that's not good for when you want to go out and play. It also makes it harder for you to fight off germs that are all around, especially at school. Being sick definitely does not feel fun and you can't play with friends. So maybe we get the applesauce cups or this bag of cherries instead of those cupcakes?"

It's worth having those conversations – it may not work every time but it starts to educate them (like the old proverb: Give a man a fish he eats for a day – TEACH him how to fish and he might just eat fewer Goldfish crackers and more apples).

Packaging very much caters to children. Does it have a cute mascot or cartoon or animal? From Ronald McDonald to the Pillsbury Doughboy to Cap'n Crunch, chances are it's a highly processed packaged food. You can tell your kids that too. "Honey, I know it looks super-fun but they are not being very truthful about how good it is for your body. Hydrogenated oils, white flour refined sugar, food colors and tons of synthetic stabilizers and preservatives eventually give your body boo-boos."

Exception: I like the Chiquita banana girl. We'll let her slide—she represents one single ingredient.

Children need to be educated. I have a friend who's husband is a doctor and when their daughter started to have solid food they didn't give her fruit, or hardly any. They went with savory foods like mashed avocado with grass-fed butter and Himalayan salt—and at seven years old that girl will tell you all the health benefits of garlic, salmon and broccoli.

Make a point to look at your groceries as they get placed on the cashiers moving belt.

CHAPTER NINE

YOUR RELATIONSHIP WITH HUNGER

Don't fear the hunger pangs. As long as you are getting enough nutrients, reaching your new weight goals will be a bit of a compromise. Before certain acting jobs where I felt I needed to lose the weight the camera put on, I learned to "embrace the hunger pangs," and took it as a sign of progress. I reiterate, I've never starved myself. I think it's impossible with my Italian upbringing, but I can be VERY disciplined with portion control. Am I hungry or am I just craving something? Maybe I'm dehydrated and need to throw back a big glass of water.

Many times, when I think I'm hungry, I'm just bored—so I get busy doing something: clean out a drawer, delete duplicate names from my contacts, hop in the car to run an overdue errand... anything but bored eating!

It's enjoyable to eat when you're hungry and then when that feeling goes away, STOP EATING. It won't be an entire plate of food, trust me. But don't punish yourself with hunger either. When your body is really hungry, give it just what it needs and no more. It only needs about 1600-

2400 calories a day. But you can easily give it 4000 calories by finishing everything on your plate when you definitely don't need it.

Even at work, you might not find yourself hungry at lunchtime and would be just as happy having a piece of turkey jerky and an apple at 3pm and then having a nice dinner. But skipping lunch around your co-workers may not be without a little drama: "Are you dieting?", "We're ordering Indian food today, that's your favorite!" You have to be prepared for these responses and shrug them off.

Back when I was in my 20s and 30s skipping a meal came with the label that you might be anorexic, but the world is very different now than it was 25 years ago and skipping lunch at the office shouldn't come across as such a shock to your co-workers.

The hunger pangs are not a bad thing—they're your body's way of saying, "Hey, I'm doing my job!" That meal you enjoyed? It's being broken down and turned into fuel, repairing, energizing, and keeping you glowing. Hunger isn't the enemy; it's just a sign your digestive system is hard at work, making magic behind the scenes. It's like when you're doing your skincare routine—sometimes you've gotta let the serum soak in before you layer on the next thing.

There's no need to freak out if you start to feel hungry and run for the snacks. Let your digestive system have its moment. Let it finish what it started, using every ounce of goodness you've already given it. Fasting isn't about going without. It's not punishment, it's self-care, it's about letting your body do its thing, uninterrupted.

Many animals will stop eating when they're unwell. It's an innate behavior — their bodies go into rest-and-repair mode, diverting energy from digestion to healing. Think of dogs or cats refusing food when they're sick. Their instincts seem to "know" that fasting helps recovery. No timers, no diet books — just nature's wisdom.

So wait until your body is REALLY ready to eat and not at the very first sign of hunger. If you feel hungry, and you look in your fridge or pantry and you can't find anything you want, you're probably not hungry. Learn to not eat by the clock. If a friend asks you if you want to eat, and you ask them what time it is, there's a good chance you're not actually hungry and that you're just relying on a time schedule. Sometimes hunger could be tiredness. Maybe you need a nap instead of a sandwich.

Trust your gut—literally! Your body is brilliant, and it knows exactly what it's doing.

IT'S EXPENSIVE TO EAT HEALTHY... OR IS IT?

We tend to think of healthy food as expensive. But when you measure and compare the nutrition you actually need, eating junk food definitely costs you more to fill you up—compared to, for example, eating one banana. You'll feel more full from that one healthy, nutrient rich banana than a bag of greasy, vitamin-deficient chips!

Growing up, my mom knew that sugary, processed foods and fast-food would weaken our immune system—not kill us, just make us more susceptible to getting sick. As a single mom working three jobs, she couldn't afford to have sick kids staying home forcing her to either miss work or pay for a sitter. So she only kept healthy simple foods in the fridge and pantry for us.

Peanut butter without sugar, whole wheat crackers, our favorite sized pickles, cans of garbanzos and refried beans, pure fruit juice popsicles, frozen bananas to make smoothies (although we called them "healthy shakes" back then), and her favorite vegetables were broccoli and garlic (garlic is often thought of as an herb or spice but it's actually a root vegetable in the same species as the onion family!). She showed us how to use the pans and how to chop onions and garlic because sautéing onion and garlic with olive oil made everything better.

For you women reading, I would suggest eating as if you were pregnant. I'd like to think that most women eat more cleanly during those months knowing they're growing a body within themselves. That thought alone will give you the discipline to make better choices. Again, we're not going for 100% clean, perfect eating 100% of the time. That's impossible. But these are little viewpoint shifts that you can take with you to help give you a little discipline to make better choices 30-40% of the time.

Imagine if this year you ate 40% healthier than the year before. Your skin would glow more, you'd feel more energized, your adrenals and immune system would strengthen. *And you'd feel more confident.* Then in the following year, you'd be eating 60% better because you saw how those choices were actually making you feel better, and look better, and were not costing you any more money or taking up any more time. You'd get to the point where food didn't control your life, it would simply be one part of it.

THE FAT-FREE ELEPHANT IN THE ROOM

I've personally never chosen fat-free. My focus has always been on nutrition and pronounceable ingredients. Your body needs healthy fats to thrive. They're like the VIPs of your diet—fueling your brain, balancing your hormones, and giving your skin that juicy, radiant glow we all crave. Fat-free products are often loaded with sneaky sugars and chemicals to make up for the flavor and texture. Your body needs the good stuff like avocados, nuts, and olive oil. It will thank you, your energy will skyrocket, and your skin will look like you just stepped off a tropical vacation.

The next time you see a "Fat-Free" label, this is probably what you will find on close inspection:

+ **Added sugar and unhealthy ingredients:** Low-fat foods are often made with added sugars, salt, and other unhealthy filler ingredients to try and make them taste better.

+ **Not calorie-free:** Fat-free foods are not calorie-free.

+ **May lack important nutrients:** These over-processed foods lack important monounsaturated fats

(Healthy oils). Your body needs dietary fat to absorb vitamins A, D, E, and K.

• **Could lead to overeating:** Low-fat foods may leave you feeling hungry, which can lead to overeating carbohydrates.

There are so many different types of fats—monounsaturated, polyunsaturated, saturated, and trans fats. Most are good in very limited amounts—*except trans fats.*

Trans Fats are basically man-made oils injected with hydrogen to keep it solid at room temperature. This manufactured ingredient is awful for your body. It's in margarine, donuts, fries (most fried food), vegetable shortening, store-bought baked goods, frosting, frozen pizza, crackers, microwave popcorn, chips, and non-dairy creamers (just to name a few).

Monounsaturated or Polyunsaturated Fats are things like olive oil, avocado, sesame seed oil, peanut and almond butter. They turn liquid at room temperature. These are definitely considered healthy fats.

And Saturated Fats, like trans fats, stay solid at room temperature *but* unlike trans fats, they are found in whole foods. They are found in salmon, red meat, chicken, pork, animal fat like lard, dairy products like butter and cream cheese as well as yogurt, eggs, and coconut oil.

So when it comes to fats:

• **Read labels carefully:** Avoid products with "partially hydrogenated oils".

- **Choose whole, unprocessed fats:** Stick to butter, coconut oil, olive oil, and nuts over margarine or vegetable shortening when cooking.
- **Limit processed foods**: If it comes in a package and has a long shelf life, it likely contains unhealthy fats.

You can look at the foods above that contain these saturated fats and deduce which ones are healthy fats. We need meat and dairy, but we need it in its purest form. Fats from fish are excellent for our skin. A roasted chicken is better than a fried chicken nugget. A tablespoon of grass-fed butter on your broccoli is far healthier than topping it with margarine (an ultra-processed oil). A real gouda cheese spread on your apple is better than the fake cheesy sauce (50% cheese, 50% artificial salty goo). A grilled burger is better than a processed meat stick. And real scrambled eggs are healthier than a Starbucks egg bite which has "powdered cellulose" (sawdust) and maltodextrin (a sugary food-additive). Not that I won't choose a Starbucks egg bite before an early plane flight instead of a sugary mochaccino, but just educating myself in knowing what's in it—and what HAS to be in it to be sold in mass quantities—makes me lower my expectations of a healthy BBA deposit.

The small amount of trans fat that might be in red meat and dairy are of less concern in its natural form. It's the unnaturally converted trans fats that are in processed food that contribute to weight gain and disease.

CHAPTER ELEVEN

DISCIPLINE, WILLPOWER, AND OTHER DIRTY WORDS

There is so much emotion wrapped in the word *self-discipline*. And yes, it's one of those "easier said than done" concepts. But I've found ways to make self-discipline as easy as eating a brownie! No, seriously, eat the brownie for God's sake! But just have one! Or just one or two bites.

Self-discipline is going to be your greatest asset to provide freedom of choice—which we all have—to improve our health.

Society has drilled into us that we need to eat for reasons other than because we are hungry. It's the multi-billion dollar diet companies and food advertisers who have taught us this at a young age, and it's been passed down. But we *can* retrain our way of looking at how, why, and when we eat.

I think one of the most common 'human elements' people struggle with is the "go big or go home" theory. The "I have to eat it all! I have no willpower," or "I deserve to eat it all." There are only two people I know who are in their 50s and 60s, are still fit, and haven't gained weight since I've known them—over 25 years! And they've stayed that way by saying, "I have to eat the whole pizza pie or the whole cake, so I just don't eat any sugar or bread. Period." They're the only two people I know who are actually THAT disciplined.

This book isn't for them. It's for people like me who enjoy ALL the food groups and the social and passionate elements that surround food.

Although we can't choose our family, we can't choose our blood type, and we can't choose what the weather will be tomorrow—we CAN choose what we put in our mouths. And to be honest, it's always been easier for me to be disciplined in the supermarket than to be disciplined at the gym.

You might think, "But what about people with health issues, etc.?" I recognize many people are obese because of their health issues. What I'm trying to say is that I'm not naturally skinny. I've been making intentional decisions about what and how I eat since I was young, and it all starts with things as simple as making those decisions before you even check out at the grocery store.

When it comes to carby-sweets, to this day I still think of that movie I saw when I was four years old, *The Fantastic Voyage*, and I envision those helpful scientists in my body, and if I finish all that ice cream they will have to form a layer of cellulite around my thighs to combat the sugars and fats. So what do I do? I lick off all the sprinkles and then throw the rest of the cone away.

When you try to apply strict discipline to what you eat, habits begin to form that won't serve you well in the flexible way of thinking. If you've gone off the wagon on a diet, the thought pattern is, "Well, what difference does it make? I already put cheese on my eggs and blew my calorie count, so I might as well eat that co-worker's birthday cake since I'm tired of punishing myself."

See how the logic in that doesn't benefit YOU? It certainly doesn't benefit your body, nor your trim mindset goal.

So if you change the diet mindset—your inner dialogue becomes more like, *Well, that extra cheese was amazing, so I'll make up the extra calories I withdrew from my BBA by having a chai tea with stevia instead of a slice of processed, sugary, inflammatory, white-flour cake.* And you can do it with an air of confidence. You make the decision from a proud, in-control viewpoint.

CHAPTER THIRTEEN

EAT THE RAINBOW

When mom said, "Eat your veggies!" she was right. A good general rule to remember is: The darker the veggie the more vitamins it holds. Arugula, spinach, and purple cabbage are staples in my diet.

My husband ironically has never been a vegetable lover. His meals are mostly beige, brown, white and yellow. The way I started getting him to have greens was when smoothies hit the scene around the year 2000... Dang, over 25 years ago! It's easy to put frozen blueberries, strawberries, water, a scoop of protein powder and 2 handfuls of raw spinach and a handful of fresh kale in a regular blender and blend that up.

For decades he's done that 4-7 times a week. It used to be his breakfast, and he used to add a banana too, but now he is minimizing his fruit sugars, especially in the morning, so he makes one mid-day or as an after-dinner dessert treat.

When we go out to eat, if he didn't make his shake he will have "his salad," which is a plain bowl of spinach and romaine lettuce – no dressing or croutons. I know, this is totally boring, but it's his way of filling his healthy BBA while catering to his own childlike palate. And for context, he's 6' 3" and still weighs about the same 185 pounds he has for the past 30+ years.

While I wish I could cook more exciting things for him, I've learned to pick my battles and guide him the best I can.

The darker the green, the brighter the red, the deeper the purple, the better it is and the more it heals you. You want to get into your body more of these colorful foods because that's what's going to help fight disease, fight infection, keep your skin plump and tight and able to heal itself.

The human body is pretty resilient and can fight off stuff if it's been put in a condition to be able to fight things off. I'll have a Pop Tart or some Doritos once a month, but I can because my system has been fed really good food, balanced out with good probiotics, toxin absorbing beans, and a lot of dark green vegetables. A standard salad at a restaurant is usually a few leaves of iceberg lettuce with some shavings of a carrot, two circle slices of a cucumber and one cherry tomato. Big whoop! You can just as easily grab a carrot and celery stalk or Persian cucumber out of your fridge and eat it while watching your favorite TV show and get 10 times the amount of nutrients.

I can't say enough about dark greens and raw vegetables. I feel it's my single most successful action for speeding up my metabolism. Veggies are primarily insoluble fiber, which means they help with keeping you regular, and they help with digestion. I always believed that if I had a brownie or a couple of slices of pizza with my husband, as long as I ate plenty of raw (or freshly cooked) vegetables before or after it, I would be in good shape. So I do.

Plenty to me means at least three full-sized carrots or four stalks of celery or half a bag of baby spinach or half a head of broccoli. If you eat out often, you may not be getting enough fresh vegetables. Sometimes I will just grab a handful of raw spinach and eat it right from the fridge or at my desk, just to get it over with, and no oily bowl to have to wash. You're done. A couple of handfuls of raw nutrient dense veggies is great for your metabolism and vital for your skin

To answer the question: Is it better to eat vegetables raw or cooked? The best answer to me is, "Whichever way you will eat it." It's like asking when is the best time to work out?" When will you do it? Or as a photographer people ask me "What is the best camera?" And I always say, "The one you are excited to pick up and USE." A healthy combination of raw and cooked is the key to vibrant health.

CHAPTER FOURTEEN

PEER PRESSURE

You are going to get pressured and "food bullied," as I have experienced a lot in my life. I constantly have people say, "Why are you ordering THAT? You don't have to diet!" And they are right. I don't diet. I make food choices that mathematically add up to more credits than debits in the BBA. Because of that cliché (but so very true) phrase:

Nothing tastes as good as healthy feels.

It can, and does, become second nature. Let's imagine for a second that you're at a restaurant with friends or family, or on a date. Maybe you don't want that guy to know you're on a diet because, if you're like me, you are tired of people giving you a hard time for making "boring" healthy choices (especially if everyone's ordering pasta and you order a salad).

What's actually happening is you're pushing the buttons of other people who wish they could be more disciplined. Knowing this allows you to be more compassionate about other people's difficulties in this very same struggle to eat healthier. When you come from a place of understanding and compassion, you can respond to them without feeling pressured and maintain your own integrity in a very unassuming, non-judgmental way.

Peer pressure doesn't always have to be people's negativity towards you. On the contrary, a celebratory baby shower is filled with tea cakes and scones, and it's almost disrespectful to NOT eat them. It can imply you are not being part of the full purpose of the celebration. That is something I have had to work through, especially when I have many friends who throw MANY parties. Being around wonderful people and platters of delicious food can really test one's discipline.

This will sound weird, and I never realized how automatically I do this until writing this book, but I always have this exterior view of my naked body when I'm going to eat an empty calorie food. I have this quick visual flash of my thighs getting more dimpled by going back for that second helping of scalloped potatoes or pumpkin pie. And because I only exercise 2-3 times a month, I can easily do the math and skip that second portion.

Instead of filling my plates with the artichoke dip and buffalo wings, I will grab a few of the gluten-free crackers next to the cheesy artichoke dip, and the celery that came with those sugary buffalo wings. This caloric math works well for my BBA. It made it a good deposit as opposed to a heftier withdrawal.

I'm also really good at taking just one bite of something—and being done with it.

I was chatting with a woman while standing over a table of desserts at a holiday party when I noticed a plastic tray of raspberry bars nearby. I said to her, "Ooo, I love me a raspberry or blueberry bar!"

She replied, "Well, those are store-bought. Try some of the homemade keto desserts over there."

I said, "I did! I tried the keto energy ball, but it was a little tasteless for me..." Then I took a knife and sliced a very thin sliver of the raspberry bar and slowly ate it, savoring all its unhealthy sweetness.

She asked, "So... how is it?"

I told her, "It's like those Italian butter cookies with the jelly filling... it's delicious."

Then she said, "Is that all you're gonna have?!"

I nodded. "Yep—because I know what the next bite will taste like: exactly the same."

She laughed and said, "Well, I can't just stop at one. I have to eat the whole thing."

I said, "Well, I would eat the whole thing if it did something good for my body. But it doesn't—so it makes me happy to at least enjoy that one awesome bite."

If I'd been feeling hungry, I would've walked over to the table with the chicken and meatballs and satisfied my hunger with protein—not dessert.

So, the one-bite method can work... when it's really just one bite. (Okay, maybe two.)

The point here is to *really* look at what is worth eating. You've actually gone to the party for the social aspect or the business networking. Remember that the stories you hear and the people you meet will ALWAYS be more meaningful and healthy for you than any pizza bite or cocktail frank. Concentrate on the social aspects at a party, and you won't get so stressed over all the bad food choices you have to restrain yourself from. Have a few tastes, but go heavier on the grapes and the chocolate covered almonds since those are a more healthy choice than a big slice of cake or tiramisu.

It all comes back to that basic food math and understanding how it all affects your BBA.

CHAPTER FIFTEEN

THE RESTAURANT CHALLENGE

Today's busy lifestyles and search for quick, convenient solutions to free up time, can lead to the pressure of trying to eat at restaurants that offer menu options and portion sizes that won't completely toxify your body. The struggle is real!

Well into my 20s and 30s, restaurant eating was still only for special occasions. I was a working actress but money was always tight. Between having an unpredictable schedule, raising my kid and working several odd jobs, date night restaurant eating was minimal. Therefore, cooking meals at home fit all my health, time, and financial goals.

But in my 40s, life got a bit more social. Business meetings in restaurants were more frequent, pushing me to adopt more easy-to-follow discipline habits than in my 20s. I know the struggle, and that's how I got very good at "doing nutritional math" and "empty calorie math" when I looked at a menu.

Furthermore, eating out isn't about filling your stomach with your entire caloric intake for the week in one night.

Which for me was very difficult because I grew up with very little money. We did grocery shopping with food stamps and decorated our house entirely from the Salvation Army and Pier One Imports when they had a big sale because my mom was an early adopter of Bohemian Style. All this to say, it's still work for me NOT to order a large platter of that nacho taco salad with more greasy ingredients than actual salad, or that country breakfast skillet pan breakfast with so many hidden nitrates and enough food to feed four people. These are "fun" and complex menu items that I didn't have growing up….but the heavier-set people in my life did. So restaurant menus get me doing nutritional and caloric math while never compromising flavor and fun.

Try Ordering Family-Style

You can order three things for four or five people. Don't ever be shy to ask, "Hey, want to split something?" They can say no. But they can also say, "Sure! I'm not that hungry anyway!" You can order the side salad instead of the French fries, and try soups as your main course. They are super excellent in winter and very satisfying in summer.

Look at the Side Order Section

This section is where I've ordered my meals for 80 percent of my restaurant visits since I was about 15—and today, I am still defaulting to the side orders. It could be a side of asparagus and a side of three meatballs. It can also be a baked potato with real butter and a side salad. You can craft a healthy meal of just two clean, simple ingredients without all the extraneous calories, sauces, sides, and portion sizes of a main entree. Just tell the waitress, "Bring me the side salad first, then the side of meatballs as my main dish, please."

Apply your peer pressure strength here too. You will get someone saying, "Is that ALL you're going to eat?" And I'll say, "Oh yea, the meatballs here are filling," or "I had a late lunch," or, "I don't eat a lot in the morning." Whatever fits. Then move on and enjoy your healthy, simple, delicious choice while enjoying the company you are with most of all!

Ditch the Menu

Unless it's a super fancy 5-star restaurant, I usually don't use the menu. I know what I want from a sandwich shop (usually a side of chili and a side salad). I know what I want from a Japanese restaurant (smoked salmon skin sushi and edamame and a seaweed salad). I know what I want from an Italian restaurant (gluten-free pasta with garlic oil and parmesan cheese or rotelli and a side of meatballs).

I'm saying this because many times the items on the menu are HUGELY CALORICALLY FILLED. They have all sorts of hidden sauces and fried fats and breads that you don't need. If you're going to a restaurant for brunch, you probably already know the ingredients they have! Now, just choose the clean ones and have them cook them for you as opposed to always doing their version. You don't need a cheese-food omelet stuffed with three types of nitrate and fatty-filled sodium-drenched meats. But two eggs scrambled with one side of meat and sliced tomatoes is a healthier, lighter choice to hash browns. Remember, they ladled a lot of margarine or liquified butter in that omelette, so customizing makes it cleaner.

When you make mashed potatoes at home you may use a whole stick of butter, but it's divided up into six to eight servings for your family dinner. In a restaurant, that same recipe might have twice as much butter and probably hydrogenated oils whipped in to make it fluffier. That same portion at a restaurant will have 2–3 times more calories than your homemade version.

Same thing with mac and cheese. It's easy for a restaurant to add inexpensive butter by the cupful to ensure a delicious creamy flavor, but if you're making it at home you have more accountability by actually seeing and controlling how much butter, oil, or cheese you are adding.

It's the same with oatmeal at a restaurant. They give you a nice serving size of brown sugar, and of course you'll dump it in. But, if you were home you'd probably stop a couple of teaspoonfuls earlier, and your palate will still enjoy that sweetness with only a moderate blood sugar spike—as opposed to the restaurant portion of syrup and sugar.

Even restaurant salads hide a lot of empty calories in processed cheeses, croutons, and fried wonton crisps. All very tasty BUT devoid of healing, healthy nutrients. I'm not saying make it "unflavorful." I'm just saying, you actually don't need as much as a commercial establishment is using. And the more you start to cook your own food, the more you will see how little additional fats and sugars you actually need to make something delicious.

The To-Go Bags

Embrace the doggy bag. It's alright to take food home. You do not have to eat everything on your plate. In Europe, they rarely even use doggy bags. The reason Europe doesn't have a lot of doggie bags is that people are staying healthy with smaller portions. There's no need for a doggie bag. But in America, everything is a bit supersized. So, remember you don't need to finish your whole meal and can actually use it as a booster to make a quick meal the next day by adding fresh veggies, beans, a scrambled egg or chicken to that leftover pasta.

Baskets of Bread and Tortilla Chips

You CAN say no to the bread. It's hard to do, I know. I rarely do it if I'm with others, but if it's just me and my husband I can, because he is celiac and can't eat it so all that warm crispy dough lands on my responsibility. When I'm with others and it's sitting on the table looking so good, I'll enjoy one delicious piece, then tell the waiter, "You can take that away, thank you."

I do the same thing with tortilla chips. My husband and I can swiftly knock off a basket of chips and the waiters usually bring another basket. Once I hit my 40s I started to tell the waiters, "No thanks, we're good." How many baskets of chips do we need to consume before, during, and after our meal?!? We're already loosening our belts or unbuttoning our jeans before the main course even comes!

I'll order a crunchy taco (corn can be less inflammatory than white flour for soft shells) and get it with grilled chicken and lettuce and cheese. The amount of cheese is so scant, it's not the end of the world. And go to town with the salsa for flavor! Sometimes I will just do a side of rice and beans—none of the sour creams and cheesy fried things.

At burger places, the lettuce wrap is getting more popular. You can even do the lettuce wrap with chicken. And don't order fries. If your hubby or friend gets them, ask for a couple and then back off. My daughter had a great idea where she would squeeze one packet of ketchup onto the plate, and however many fries she got from that she would eat, and then throw the rest away.

And my "healthy" soda hack is to do ¾ club soda (soda water) and ¼ soda of choice. I don't like diet drinks due to the synthetic sugars, so I do ¾ soda water and ¼ regular. You can also ask the drive through person to make your drink this way for you.

CHAPTER SIXTEEN

AIRPLANES

Say "yes" to the water. And "no" to sugary or alcoholic drinks. Planes are already a very dehydrating environment and with varying cabin pressure and about 50% recirculated air. Don't compound the error with sugar and booze. Club soda will become your best friend on flights. And yes, you will end up having to get up and go pee, but it becomes DOUBLY GOOD because both you and the person sitting next to you get the healthy advantage of standing up after hours of sedentary inactivity to take a much needed 'free-exercise' walk to the bathroom. Then, while you are back there, chat with the flight attendant and stretch your calves, bounce up and down on your toes for a few moments. Don't worry who's watching. You'd be surprised. You will actually inspire at least one person with this healthy habit.

Remember, every piece of movement helps when you're not going to the gym every day!

Say no to the free snack…the only ones that are worth it for your body are the nuts and the healthier grain bars. Otherwise skip it. That's a tough one for me because I always make use of the free facility BUT if it's empty destructive calories, I know I'm doing my body a favor by saying no. If it's a long flight and you didn't bring a healthy snack, say yes to *just one* of the two or three times they offer it.

Once more I want to emphasize, water water water, to satiate the desire to snack. Think of it this way: You're captive in a dehydrated metal tube for 3-6 hours (already not the healthiest environment), so don't make matters worse for yourself with dehydrating sodas, booze, empty carbs and sugar. Save those "treats" for a more celebratory time.

Airplane Skincare Tip:

Sit by the window and control the window. Keep it closed to protect your skin. Bring facial misting (with my company's *Blue Tansy Hydrating Face Mist*) to spritz during the flight and if you're a real baller, give yourself a sheet mask.

CHAPTER SEVENTEEN

LIVING THE LIFESTYLE

Your body is set up to survive. It has natural urges. Though they can get exaggerated, and even masked or manipulated by advertising and imagery of a rich gluttonous life—lots of food covering your plate and the need to finish it all because, "There are people starving in Africa..."

Once you listen to your body, whether it wants a burger or steamed broccoli, and you are hungry, don't deprive yourself. Too many of those depravations and "can't-haves" backfire, and that's when binge eating and "I deserve this" start to take over.

With this one mindset, my mom really started to lose the weight she had gained over the years after my brother's death.

When I visited her, I saw her eating straight from a carton of Häagen-Dazs—like she'd done for years. But this time, I watched her take three bites, close it, and walk back to the kitchen.

I yelled out, "Are you putting that back in the freezer?!"

"Yes!" she said.

I was amazed. Then she told me, "The fourth bite tastes just like the fifth and sixth, so I stop at the fourth and put it back for another time."

I felt like Henry Higgins and she was Eliza Doolittle from *My Fair Lady*: "By George, I think she's got it!"

I've found that whenever I'm fully immersed in an activity I love, I am not thinking about food. I'm sure you have times in your life where you may have been helping a friend decorate their house for a baby shower, and you're making flower arrangements and moving furniture and cutting tea sandwiches (or whatever your version of creating a beautiful party is), and suddenly it's four-thirty in the afternoon and all you had eaten was a cup of coffee in the morning and a gulp of a protein shake you made, but forgot to take with you. And guess what? You didn't die. You didn't faint. Your body had an inadvertent fast and was very occupied using all the nutrients from the day before and then had a relaxing time burning fat and increasing cellular regeneration.

Live in the present. Don't obsess about the next meal. There's more to life than eating. It's just a small part of the day.

How I Eat

Growing up, we couldn't afford a lot of meat, so I was raised with lots of rice and beans and great Mexican food in Los Angeles. But the summers I spent with my Italian grandparents in New York were filled with lots of fresh fish we would catch as well as lots of pasta. Because of their backyard garden, we would eat countless vegetables: Zucchini, tomatoes, green beans, fennel, cucumbers, you name it. These few items were either sauteed with fresh onions and garlic to put atop of pasta or finely chopped for a crunchy salad to accompany a fresh thin fillet of seasoned, breadcrumbed, olive oil-fried flounder.... I'm drooling and slightly teary eyed at the very thought of these delicious pleasure moments. To this day I consume a lot of vegetables, and a lot of fats like nuts, butters, oils, and beans.

Making a mini pizza in your own kitchen from a slice of whole grain toast or some crusty french bread will always taste better, have more nutrients, more fiber and be lower in calories than store bought mini frozen pizzas. That also includes the choices from diet brands and even "healthy" organic brands. Premade food usually has added sugars, salts and preservatives that you don't need. While making your own you can use higher quality ingredients: Olive oil and mineral rich Celtic or Himalayan salt. So if you're craving a delicious pizza treat, take some Ezekiel bread, some shaved parmesan, low-fat mozzarella, or even cottage cheese, tomato, a shake of basil and bake it up... Mama Mia, that sounds so tasty!

At the Office

I've been a self-employed artist all of my life (with two years, 2005-2007, spent as a talent agent in a Hollywood office). But now at 59, I run a skincare company and show up to my desk job every morning at 8:30am without fail.

I'm officially a "9 to 5er," and my days of working from home as an actress and photographer are no more.

So now I am forced to get creative in our mini staff kitchen. I actually brought in a single burner that plugs in for every time I want to sauté some chicken sausages or chili, or heat up a quinoa stir fry I made the night before. Jars of almond butter and ak-mak crackers, cans of tuna fish, condiments like mayonnaise and mustard, bottles of olive oil and balsamic vinegar and even lemon juice are always stocked. My mom banned microwaves from our home growing up, and so I've always preferred the speed of cooking on a stove top—it's evenly and quickly heated and radiation-free!

Part of my purpose in writing this book is to share how easy it is to eat healthy while also not spending a lot of money. So, even when I'm in a hotel, or on location filming, I make sure to always have a cutting board and a knife because I can make healthy snacks and salads from celery and peanut butter, cucumber tomato salads with feta cheese, etc. You can even buy cooked hard boiled eggs in convenience stores and mash them up with a little packet of mayo, mustard and a shake of tabasco. Don't forget to haul a fork with you too!

A few years ago, I had forgotten a fork and was eating a baked potato from a Wendy's drive-thru with my hands. I was starving, driving to an audition, and I posted about the crazy situation on Facebook. A soap opera fan saw the post and sent me a camping utensil to keep in my car so I'd never have to do that again! And let me tell you, I've used that tool several times. Moral of the story, never forget about the silverware in your food emergency kit!

At the office, I'm a big Tupperware user. Most often I try to stick to glass Tupperware. I like to use small containers for storing dressing for salads or for dipping raw veggies. Remember, we are packing these healthy food items to take with us to work so that we can indulge a bit at that upcoming birthday party or that trip to Europe we've been saving up for. You have to earn those calories by making those super clean choices every moment you can. It's a little bit like how I get excited to deposit a paycheck into my bank account. It's the same excitement I get for choosing light and clean food at a restaurant and having no fried foods for four days in a row. Then I've earned that pizza and half a slice of tiramisu.

It's never about depriving yourself. It's controlling your destiny from a healthy, responsible, loving viewpoint about your body. It's treating your body always like a newborn baby and giving it what you know your blood cells and adrenals want and need to grow and heal. NOT what your taste buds want. Those are two different things. Though, every once in a while you can feed your taste buds. The irony of it is that the more you start to shift your mindset to the simpler, whole-food way of eating, you'll crave those healthy items more. You won't feel like, "little poor me." You'll feel proud, sexy and in control of that gorgeous vessel we call our body!

My Pantry

I realize in a household with kids it's almost impossible to not have sweet cakey snacks in your pantry, but there is a balance. There are healthier substitutes you can get and their younger bodies can metabolize the extra calories a bit faster than our older bodies. So in order to not tempt **my own** tastebuds with buying desserts that I had a weakness for like carrot cake and jelly donuts, which my daughter and husband were not as much of a fan of, I would get them treats that I could pass on.

This is a very small discipline step and is easier than having to hit a gym every day. Even if the organic carrot cake or those jelly donuts are "buy one get one free", it's primarily empty calories that only **you** will be eating. I justify this "Act of Deprivation," which is actually a "Gift of Health" to myself, by realizing I always have some upcoming birthday party, baby shower, wedding or grand opening to go to where there's probably going to be some junk food there and I can indulge in a treat.

This leads me to another healthy hack: **I don't like to eat junk food by myself. To me that's such a waste of calories.** If I'm going to kill my adrenal glands, I at least want to have the joy and company of a social experience. When I'm by myself at home and I'm working on my computer, I'm not going to go for the junk food, but I will say yes to it at a social function. And even then, it's just going to be a couple of bites and I'll just toss it. The trash can's feelings do not get hurt when you feed it, and your abs will thank you.

Puny Portions...Good or Bad?

Make your salad bowl bigger! As a rule of thumb I try to use large bowls to eat my salads in and smaller plates for carbs, protein, and desserts. I have made videos where I show the amount of veggies in a restaurant salad or a veggie side and then how much you can put in a homemade salad or your own veggie stir fry. The difference is astounding.

A few shavings of a carrot atop a side salad doesn't really qualify as having a serving of carrots. But if you are home you can shave one whole carrot and that will add to your BBA. Or faster still, crunch on it like Bugs Bunny while you are making your green salad. I'm not a fan of chunks of carrots in a salad, so I eat them ahead of time and get them over with.

I have a lot of big bowls that make me happy. I'll even find them at thrift stores or garage sales. When I'm preparing my salad I'm inspired to "super size" it by the size of my bowl.

Nothing wrong with feeling satisfied when you're done with your salad. You'll also be less likely to eat those high calorie foods.

Leftovers

Whether it's from a restaurant or from your own kitchen, giving a new spin on food can be super delicious and save you time and money. I give Chinese food leftovers a healthy boost by adding more chopped veggies and scrambled egg and even a healthy garlic clove to the leftover fried rice, or add fresh zucchini and onion to any leftover stir fry. Even left over protein, like steak and chicken, can have a second life brought into another culture like turning an American steak or chicken leftover dinner into Mexican fajita stir fry—slice the meat and sauté with bell peppers and onions and a dash of chili powder or salsa sauce.

Sugar

As I mentioned, when I was 12 that nutritionist told me "sugar gives you wrinkles and can make you sick." Oddly enough, that stayed with me. It doesn't mean I've avoided sugar successfully my whole life. But this awareness of what it can do when not "used properly" like when it is paired with proteins, has helped me to navigate through the abundance of sugar-ladened foods.

Here's a term most of you probably know: *Glycemic Index*. It is a ranking of foods based on how they affect your blood sugar on a scale from 1-100. 70+ is high, 56-69 is medium, and 55 and under is low. **And Low is good**.

Limit drinking fruit juices like apple and orange juice. One glass is like six oranges or apples but without the fiber and just the sugars. That converts to fat. Blended fruit in a smoothie at least gives you the benefits of the whole fruit.

My go-to drink has always been some iced tea – if you need a pinch of sweetener like stevia, monk fruit or simple syrup (liquid sugar) go for it. It's still healthier than any of the sugary food colored drinks out there.

My go to sweeteners are, enzyme-rich local honey, maple syrup, monk fruit and coconut sugar for baking.

I could go on and on about sugar and how refined white flour and minute rice and tortilla chips spike your glucose levels but I'm not giving medical advice. I only want to make you aware in a very practical and tolerant way that sugar is hidden in so many foods and is advertised as a shining star. When in actual fact it's quite the dirty little villain.

Mmmmmmm....yummmm.....Bread

If you're trying to trim down, it's good to cut back on this. Now, mind you there are times where you will be at a restaurant known for its wood-furnace baked organic breads or focaccias…THAT'S when you want to have the splurge. Not the lame, tasteless nutritionless bread at Subway or the corner deli or supermarket party platter. White bread has a glycemic index of 70 or more and wheat bread comes in at 55-60. You're better off doing the salad version or lettuce wrap.

Do you know about Ezekiel bread? You can get it in most regular supermarkets. It's made from sprouted grain. It's not gluten free but it's the lowest glycemic index bread on the market at 36. Wow! Pass the butter, baby!

I grew up in 70s and 80s, and granola was quite popular but also quite high in sugars…but these days granolas are made with less sugars and more superfoods and anti-oxidants like chia, and flax seeds and dried cherries and blueberries, along with a base of oats and nuts. It's a great breakfast with some Greek yogurt or a grapefruit. Maybe even a couple strips of bacon! Aww, man. I will confess to you; I was a vegetarian for 7 yrs… but I still had bacon.

My View on Sweet vs Savory

Listen, I get it—sweet foods, even the so-called "keto-friendly" ones, feel like the ultimate treat. But here's the deal: Your brain doesn't care if it's sugar-free. Sweetness is sweetness, and it lights up the same "Gimme more!" pathway, leaving you reaching for another bite, and another, and… Well, you get the picture.

But here's a better idea: Swap that sweetness for savory delights that satisfy and nourish without setting off those dessert sirens—think herbed hummus, crispy kale chips, or a hearty, spiced bone broth. Embrace the savory side of life. Try roasted veggies, roasted almonds, or a creamy avocado mash—foods that satisfy without setting off the dessert alarm. It's a little shift with big rewards. Trust me, the more you lean into those rich, savory flavors, the quieter those sugar cravings will become, and your brain won't miss the sweetness. You'll feel grounded, balanced, and totally in charge of your plate.

Soup Symphony: Start with a Can, End with a Masterpiece

Here's a great food hack for you: Think of a can of soup like the steady beat of a drummer—simple, reliable, setting the foundation. But a great meal, like great jazz, is all about improvisation!

The Veggie Solo: Toss in fresh spinach, chopped bell peppers, or shredded carrots for a crisp, colorful melody.

The Protein Riff: Shred some rotisserie chicken, crack in an egg, or add a handful of beans for a hearty groove.

73

The Herb Crescendo: A sprinkle of fresh basil, a dash of thyme, or a swirl of lemon zest takes the flavor up an octave.

The Finishing Flourish: A dollop of Greek yogurt, a drizzle of olive oil, or a shake of red pepper flakes gives it that final, flavorful baseline.

Suddenly, your basic can of soup transforms into a flavorful, free-spirited jam session in a bowl.

Take Care of Your Skin

When we see a woman with glowing and radiant skin, we usually think "What products is she using?" And that goes for healthy teeth, clear white eyes, a toned fit body, and shiny or thick hair. We usually assume, and even hope, that it's all the result of one or two products. But an all over radiant health comes predominantly from what you put in your body, the foods you eat and the beverages you consume. Sometimes I wish it wasn't the case, but as a young teenager growing up with a single working mom and not a lot of money, we couldn't afford gym memberships, dermatologist and spa trips—even doctor and dentist trips were taken on a very limited basis because of our monthly bills.

So much of what we see as aging on our faces is unrepaired damage to our body. And that's because the body hasn't been given the nutrition to help bolster normal cell turnover and hormonal decline that occurs over time. So much of my beauty regimen actually has nothing to do with the products on my bathroom shelves *but with what is in my refrigerator.*

My skin doesn't care how many vitamin C serums I own if my fridge looks like a college dorm after finals week. The glow is not just in that jar; it's also in the kale, the berries, and the water you're skipping for soda. You have to stock your fridge like your skin depends on it—because it does!

As the founder of a skincare line, I absolutely apply the same healthy standard for a holistic approach to beautiful skin as I do with nutrition. My company's motto is *Using Mother Nature to Stop Father Time®*.

Now, there are many benefits to DIY skin care remedies and routines but not everything from your kitchen cupboards is in a molecular state to be able to be effective to your skin's epidermal layer. Your face has pores but those pores don't have teeth and a digestive system. So that is why I created formulas that have a high concentration of Mother Nature's active ingredients but are scientifically crafted in a way that's highly effective and recognizable to your microbiome.

The way I choose the foods I eat is how I choose the ingredients for my products: More of the good and little to none of the inert and harmful. It's true that there are certain "filler ingredients" needed to deliver certain vitamins and antioxidants in your skincare products, but companies have taken advantage of the public who can't decipher long winded product labels to actually know what it is they are putting on their face. Most drugstore brands will "trace in" a popular ingredient like jojoba oil or a peptide. This means they put in the lowest amount allowable. So it won't even be effective. But the creators save money this way and can still make the "Label Claim" when what you are actually buying is primarily a jar of microplastics and synthesized cheap oils and emulsifiers.

Grrr… it makes me so mad.

Skin health has always been very important to me, especially having looked at it through a close lens for decades. My personal skin care regimen was simple and inspired by my great-grandmother. My personal face cream was my "secret weapon." It had simple, practically edible, ingredients.

I want every beauty product I use to make my face feel something because then I know it's DOING something. We know feeding our bodies healthy organic foods helps our guts and hormones to create a strong intestinal environment to fight off toxins. It's the same with what you "feed your face." Because after all, your skin deserves the same respect as your stomach.

I want to always use ingredients my body recognizes to create products that never compromise health for beauty. Companies have profits to make and they need their products to last a long time sitting on the shelf or even in the freezer. I have seen firsthand how healthy formulas have to be modified to last on shelves in hot warehouses. I've seen formulas get diluted with more micro-plastic liquids because they have incredibly long shelf lives and feel really good but do not add any nutrients to your skin. Jars full of dead and liquefied plastics and petroleum are being sold in the skincare world by the millions, because they can be made in large quantities and are very profitable.

To put it simply, and in terms of food, small batches of freshly picked peaches are more costly than a can of corn syrup-laden peaches. BUT that fresh peach is vastly more alive and healthy for your beautiful body.

I create skincare where the formulas are more "Kale and avocado, and less iceberg lettuce and hydrogenated oil." You see, iceberg lettuce will not harm you, but it absolutely won't give your body the nutrition it needs to reach your health goals. I want my skincare to work fast with nutrient dense formulas, not watered down in microplastics. And I apply my same rules of nutrition to skincare as I would with feeding my body the foods it needs to survive well and happily.

CHAPTER EIGHTEEN

VEGGIES WITH BENEFITS

According to a publishing[1] from Harvard Medical School, a total of five servings per day of fruits and vegetables can provide us with the strongest health benefits.

My husband and I have extremely different eating habits. As he says "I live to eat and he just eats to live." He doesn't like spices or flavors and I can't get enough of them. He loves plain and dry sandwiches, and I love flavorful spicy stir frys. I mention this because you *can* have different palates from your spouse and family and still enjoy meals together. There's no reason to blame your kids or husband for why you are eating nachos and lunchables everyday.

As I mentioned, he doesn't like salads, or any salad dressings, but since he has many other good qualities I don't kick him out of bed (haha!). He *has* learned about the *BBA*, so he also adopted this healthy habit. He grabs a medium handful of spinach and eats it raw before he eats his lunch sandwiches (turkey, chicken or hamburger...plain, no mayo, no special sauces, and sadly, no veggies). He also doesn't buy soda for the house and only occasionally will order one as a treat at a pizza place or stadium.

Finely chop and shred your veggies. My grandmother used her cheese grater—you know the one that looks like a tall, fat four-sided building? And she would grate carrots and zucchini and hearts of romaine and splash red wine vinegar with a tablespoon of mayonnaise and sometimes a little grated parmesan. It was savory, zesty, crunchy and full of nutrients.

Good salad dressings are worth the investment. Cheap salad dressings can taste institutional and more like preservatives and corn syrup. A good quality dressing with real olive oil, fresh herbs and artisan vinegars can completely make you crave that romaine lettuce or field greens salad. So look for the ones in the healthier section and glance at the ingredient list!

Don't buy salad dressing with high fructose corn syrup or a bunch of unpronounceable diglycerides. Just expect to pay 2 dollars more than you are comfortable with but realize you're saving easily 75 bucks on what you'd pay for all those salads that you'll be able to make with this dressing at home.

Take a minute to look at the ingredients that have flavors that make you fall in love with chopped salads. And if you can make raw cabbage (purple or green), kale or arugula lettuce taste delicious, you're ahead of the game And of course, making your own salad dressings is one of the most health-empowering skills to acquire. Trust me, after buying several yummy ones, you start to memorize the ingredients and the flavor profiles and then you can closely recreate these salad dressings as they are easy, cheap and delicious!

I'm always looking for more ways to get more greens into my diet that way. So, what I'll do is I'll steam something like chicken sausages—the precooked free-range sausages. And then I'll find all the greens I have in my refrigerator—whether it's green onions, spinach, kale, zucchini, or even lettuce. Once the sausages are steamed, and they're usually cooked anyway when you buy them, throw all of your greens in it. It wilts and it's done super fast.

My grandfather was not a fan of salads, and most food for that matter, from restaurants. He said the salads were not cut up enough and the lettuce flapped in his face: "Chop that shit up!" I think he single-handedly contributed to the chopped salad trend that finally arrived in the 80s.

When my grandfather made fresh clam sauce, he would scrape all the meat from the clam and finely chop it. Then, he threw it in a hot pan of simmering olive oil with chopped garlic and a handful of fresh cut parsley. He'd simmer this down, then add the linguine, and sometimes a bit of butter, and stir until the clams all stuck to each strand of pasta with the bits of parsley and garlic.

One time, when I was about 15 years old we were at a restaurant with him, and he ordered linguine and clam sauce. Well, the waiter brought out a plate with the linguini pasta in a pool of liquid broth and about 10 steamed open clam shells looking up at him with a few flakes of parsley. He looked down at it and said, "I'm paying for this and they are making ME do all the work? Fa Napoli!" He got up and went into the kitchen and was there for 10 minutes. And, of course, returned with the chef smiling, arms on their shoulders. He had his finely chopped clams sautéed in the olive oil and garlic and parsley to get all the flavor to stick to each bite. You see, my family preferred an easy and fully flavorful eating experience over a beautiful presentation.

So go ahead—chop it, season it, and make it yours. It doesn't need to look like it came from a five-star foodie's Instagram.

CHAPTER NINETEEN

ONION AND GARLIC

Alright, my friends—let's talk about two of the most powerful, flavor-packed, health-boosting ingredients on the planet: garlic and onions. I'm talking about real, fresh garlic and onions—not the powdered stuff—because these little gems are LOADED with benefits your body will love. And yes, it's totally inspired by my Italian roots, where every meal starts with that irresistible sizzle of garlic and onions in olive oil. Healthy eating should NEVER be boring.

So why should you be eating them every day? Because they're nature's medicine! Garlic is a powerhouse for your immune system, fights inflammation, and can even help keep your blood pressure in check. Onions? They're packed with antioxidants, support your gut with prebiotics, and can help balance blood sugar. It's like a mini spa day for your insides!

And don't even THINK about saying you "don't know how" to add them to your meals—because it's SO EASY!

- **Start your morning right:** Add sautéed onions and garlic to your scrambled eggs or omelet. Boom—flavor and health in one bite.

- **Toss it in a salad:** Raw red onions add crunch and detoxifying power to any fresh salad.

- **Roast 'em up:** Chop onions and whole garlic cloves, toss them with olive oil, and roast alongside your veggies or chicken. Your house will smell like heaven.

- **Soup magic:** Every good soup, stew, or sauce starts with onions and garlic. It's the foundation of deliciousness!

My husband is celiac and can't have wheat but he has a favorite frozen pizza that he likes to eat once a week. The only way I can justify eating it is by crushing four large garlic cloves and smashing them in a little bowl of olive oil with some ground chili pepper and Himalayan salt. Then I scoop that on all my slices. At least I know I am getting the life-giving benefits of that raw garlic and not just the rice/tapioca flour crust with some cheese and a schmear of tomato sauce.

This beautiful and very wealthy Russian friend of mine was doing a cleanse of sorts. I was in a hotel room with her and she ordered room service. Her meal was a huge plate of sautéed onions and a shredded cabbage salad with apple cider vinegar dressing. It just reminded me that onions don't just have to be a flavor enhancer. They are a low calorie, super high nutritional food all on their own. Load them up raw in a salad or chopped up liberally in soups and sautés.

How many times do people say "no onion"? Every time they say no onion they're saying, "I want less vitamin content in my food. I want less antioxidants and superfoods because I don't want the onion breath." Ironically a healthy gut will absorb that flavor and you'll be fine. It's the coffee and cigarette breath they should be curtailing. So, say "yes" to those healthy onions (and then yes to a breath mint).

Eat more garlic. Eat more onions. Your taste buds will be happy, your gut will be thriving, and your body will be thanking you for years to come!

CHAPTER TWENTY

TEA, MY NOT-SO-SECRET WEAPON

Did you know: All the popular caffeinated teas from Black, Darjeeling, Oolong, Green, English Breakfast, Earl Grey, Ceylon, Jasmine Pearl, and White tea are all from the same plant. Yep. ALL from ONE plant: The Camellia Sinensis shrub.

The only difference about all these teas is how they are processed and fermented. You can break it down into three main categories: White Tea, Green Tea, and Black Tea. White being the least caffeinated, Black being the most.

White tea is from the young buds of the Camellia Sinensis shrub. It undergoes the least processing. The leaves are hand picked and usually should still have fine white hairs. They are then dried quickly to prevent oxidation. White tea has a highest concentration of catechins and antioxidants which support the immune system.

Green tea leaves are dried and heated to halt oxidation and keep the leaves green to maintain the nutritional components of the plant. Green tea leaves are not exposed to oxygen so they are considered unoxidized and retain the green color that gives them a refreshing taste profile.

The most nutrient-dense green tea is Matcha Tea. Matcha is processed and created by the Camellia Sinensis shrub being shielded from the sun for 20-30 days before harvesting. This creates more chlorophyll production in the plant turning the leaves an even darker green. These leaves are rich in amino acids and polyphenols. The stems and stalks are removed and then the leaves are crushed to a powder. This also makes matcha usually more caffeinated and antioxidant rich than regular green tea because you are consuming the actual plant. Matcha naturally has a slightly bitter grassy taste and is well sweetened with a bit of honey or monk fruit.

Please avoid the matcha from famous coffee drive-thrus as their ice blended matcha has 51% refined sugar, dextrin (more sweetener) and vegetable oil and you can't get it unsweetened because it's in their premade powder. Best to order a cappuccino as you don't need 30 grams of sugar and 200-300 calories with a large matcha frappuccino with whipped cream. Very clever marketing to the tune of 10 billion dollars since they introduced the matcha drink. And I won't even get into whether it's real matcha which needs care in harvesting and lots of shade or if it's sencha tea which stays in full sun.

Black tea leaves are green tea leaves that have been oxidized...meaning exposed to oxygen and then dried. This oxidation gives them a bolder flavor but also removes some of the phytonutrients. The leaves are withered, and rolled to release enzymes, fully oxidized, and then dried. Black tea supports heart health, aids digestion, and boosts focus due to its theaflavins and higher caffeine content.

Wild right?!! All these uses from one mighty plant.

There are two other caffeinated tea plants: Herba Matte and Yaupon Holly. Not very well known but you might win this question at a trivia game.

I love steeping my own jasmine pearl tea leaves. I have loose tea steeping pots that make it easy to brew, strain and serve. It has caffeine but not as much as coffee and is less acidic on your system. It also contains fat-burning phyto-chemicals.

The rest of the so-called teas are herbal "teas." They are herbal non-caffeinated plants and flowers: Peppermint, Rooibos (red African plant), Chamomile, Licorice, lemongrass and herbal infusions like Bengal spice. Chai Tea contains black caffeinated tea leaves along with added spices…but unless noted, it is a caffeinated tea.

There is definitely something to be said for the gut regulating properties of tea and I have to attribute it to one of the several reasons I've maintained a flat tummy.

CHAPTER TWENTY-ONE

RETHINKING SWEETNESS

Growing up I did not have the average American family routine because my mom worked at night and my brother and I didn't have a dad. We were close with all of our apartment neighbors so my mom felt safe, and we were. Because of that, we usually ate dinner in front of the TV and then went into our respective bedrooms where we either argued over who would get the phone to call our friends or listened to the radio and played records. We didn't do dessert. I remember rarely having cakes and cookies in the house. My mom knew they would weaken our immune system making us more susceptible to sickness, which was time consuming and expensive for a single mom.

Around the 2000s, sugar-free, dairy-free, gluten-free recipes really hit the recipe blogs of the internet, and I usually saw yo-yo dieters and women who struggled to lose weight being the ones to make those recipes. I was raised with a more Mediterranean view of, "Order the cannoli, you don't have to finish it all—or just spend more time gardening tomorrow."

We did make desserts as a family on special occasions. I've baked many boxes of Betty Crocker cookies and brownies using olive oil or avocado oil instead of trans-fat filled shortening, palm oil, vegetable (corn) oil, or canola (rapeseed) oil. My mom knew that buying them already made from Costco for easy snacking wouldn't do us any favors.

So when I became a wife and mother, by default I also became the family nurse, and nutritionist. I knew the consequences of easy-to-eat sweets in the cupboards so I never had that kind of food on my weekly shopping list.

My husband, daughter and I would usually end dinner by talking, doing homework, a DIY home project or watching a movie with some popcorn. Dessert wasn't part of the normal eating routine. I also knew there was always going to be some party or gathering during the week where you can be sure there would be sugary sweets to tempt everyone with.

I saved my calories for those special outings and kept the sweets down to a minimum at home. Fruit was readily available, applesauce without added sugar, even canned fruit has more healthy fiber than a sleeve of Oreo cookies. Find that balance.

Have you ever blended up a frozen banana? Delicious! A warm cup of chai tea with cream? Late at night I might scoop a couple of teaspoons of unsweetened fruit preserves with nut butter, no bread needed!

When ordering ice cream, I am quite happy with the lower calorie and lower fat option of sorbets. Lemon and raspberry—a very light alternative. Sliced apples and drizzled honey with some shakes of cinnamon can be put in a frying pan with a little water and a touch of butter and sauté that and you will have a warm, satisfying apple pie snack with hardly any calories and all those ingredients are actually good for you. You can also beat some real whipping cream—so much healthier than what's in the spray can.

Many times when you are craving something sweet, you should try drinking some water first. Some people like it more than others. I wish I loved it. But I don't really. It's a chore for me, whereas my husband drinks glasses and glasses of water on his desk from morning to night. If it's not your favorite thing, find out how best you'll drink your water: Is it carbonated? Is it with a splash of lemon or electrolyte powder? Is it room temperature out of a glass bottle? (that's me). Is it out of a ginormous Stanley cup? I always make sure to have a large amount of water whenever I have to drive somewhere because it's the perfect healthy multitasking activity.

Also if you are craving sweets, you might need a little protein. So having healthy beef or turkey sticks around, nuts, or keeping some hard boiled eggs in a bowl in your fridge are a healthier deposit to your BBA than a half a pint of Häagen-Dazs.

CHAPTER TWENTY-TWO
MY CHINESE NEIGHBORS

In third grade my parents divorced, and my mom, brother and I moved to an apartment in North Hollywood, California. I became best friends with the Chinese neighbors who also owned a famous Chinese restaurant called Genghis Khan. Actors like Farrah Fawcett, Vince Van Patten and Sally Kirkland would frequent this place.

I spent my weekends earning a few dollars chopping onions and garlic, making wontons, peeling the tough skin from broccoli stems, shredding cabbage and folding napkins. This is where I learned how to sauté fresh vegetables with plenty of flavor–they didn't really do a traditional steam of the vegetables, but didn't deep fry them either. They used giant metal woks and added liquid seasoning like broths, oyster sauces, soy sauce and splashes of water while constantly mixing the veggies, fish, chicken and scrambled eggs. The flavors seeped into every morsel.

To this day I'm the only person I know who strips the tough skin off the broccoli trunk and chops those green healthy circles to sauté with the heads. They didn't waste a thing, just like my Italian family.

The One Pan Sauté

I have very limited memories of my mom baking meals or making casseroles for dinner growing up. Then again, she worked the graveyard shift from 4pm to 2am at General Motors from the time I was in 4th grade until I was 30. So I was the one in charge of making dinners for me and my brother almost every night.

My love and skill of the one-pan sauté is deeply rooted in and inspired by my decade of growing up in my friend's Chinese restaurant. Sautéing became the fastest way to cook all the ingredients my mom bought for me to use throughout the week. They always had a rice steamer filled with warm sticky rice so my mom bought one of those to use. When quinoa hit the scene as a popular grain/seed in the early 90s, I started to mix it with my rice in the rice cooker to cut down on so much starch. The quinoa cooked as fast as the rice and was less inflammatory, gluten free, and helped with blood sugar levels. It's also full of fiber, and has protein benefits because it contains all nine essential amino acids.

So almost every night I would sauté zucchini, green onion, regular onion and mushrooms and mix that with the quinoa, even scrambling an egg for more protein. These ingredients were all perfect for our breakfast, lunch or dinner.

CHAPTER TWENTY-THREE

THE MARRIED LIFE MEALS

After getting married, I did not change my eating habits to fit my husband's lifestyle/eating habits. I must admit, I had seen and heard many stories of couples gaining weight early in their marriage over the "bliss of new love." I decided this wouldn't happen to us.

My husband has a very different way of eating than me. He was raised with a meat and potatoes, Irish-American, style diet. His mom gave them vegetables but they were always from a can. So when I came into his life it took me years to introduce real, fiber-filled vegetables.

Our meals, still to this day, look VERY different from one another. He doesn't like spice or seasoning or sauces and he has zero adventurousness about "trying new foods". He is also a celiac. His mother and brother were diagnosed in the late 1970s back in Massachusetts when no one really knew what gluten was. His mother started buying gluten-free flour from mail-order catalogues.

One summer, in 1975, I was staying with my grandparents in Queens. I was 10 years old. My grandfather was

50 at the time and had been diagnosed with diabetes. He didn't want to stop eating his treats all-together. So he had my grandmother freeze his Entenmann's cake. I remember asking, "Pop Pop why are you freezing the cake?" And he said, "Because I don't really like it when it's frozen, so I eat less of it." After about eight years he started to love it, but he had seven good years of discipline.

It's the same with my husband now. I will bake him the gluten-free cookies he loves, and he is a disciplined sweet snacker and he also freezes them—because he likes them that way—but he knows I don't love a frozen cookie as much as a room temperature one. Also, they are harder to eat frozen and you don't see them as easily because they're in the freezer... usually hidden."

Although my husband can't have wheat, he still consumes a lot of starches like rice, corn, potatoes and pizza, and basic proteins like burgers, steak, and plain white chicken. I'm always wanting him to get greens so he puts them in a smoothie he makes 4-6 days a week. He stays trim and is able to still play soccer with his "over 60 league" and that kind of movement is priceless...at any age!

As a couple, we do DIY projects at home more than restaurant-centric dinners. Our activities together never really involved dining at a restaurant. They were long walks around the city. Time together has always been more about creating or building things. Cooking separate meals has never been an issue for 35 years. His food has always been super easy to make as he only likes five foods and almost no flavor. So the time saved has always gone towards me and my daughter's more adventurous salads and stir fries. Even as an empty nester now, I make his plain, dry turkey sandwich, with a slice of cheese, a side of kettle chips and ice water, and then make my tuna fish salad with chopped red onion, scallions, celery, fresh lemon juice, and a scoop of mayo. All chopped finely then scooped onto a bed of spinach or arugula with an iced green tea.

Lickety split, no need to compromise, and more focus on time spent together rather than the food we eat.

CHAPTER TWENTY-FOUR

MOVE!

"Movement is a privilege. If you can move, you must!"
– Kacy Duke

Kacy was my neighbor when I lived in Manhattan and a very busy celebrity fitness expert and owner of *Age Defying Physique*. At 65 years old she had the body of a fit 35-year-old and wasn't starving herself or pumping iron seven days a week. She ate balanced and clean and whenever we treated ourselves to a slice of strawberry cake from our favorite french bakery or a slice of pizza from the Highline Pizzeria, it wasn't until we had clocked a couple of miles of walking through the city. It's all about Balance and Movement.

Balance keeps you sane and Movement keeps you healthy.

Gyms are glorious places. And absolutely should be used especially if you have a free one in your home, apartment complex or one that is walking distance. To me that's a sign that you MUST use it. If you have a budget for a personal trainer even once a week that's a good way to start a routine and learn to push yourself and be accountable. The first and only time I had a personal trainer was for six months, three times a week, from 7-8am for 40 bucks total for both me and my husband. His gym was a 3-minute drive down our block and we were home by 8:05am, feeling amazing. That trainer moved out of state so we decided to start buying some of our own equipment in our office once we learned a few exercise routines and how much we could push our bodies.

Nowadays, I have some friends that I can meet with in the morning to go for a long walk or meet at our office gym because it's hard for me to just do it on my own. I've never been that motivated but I AM very social, and I'm always amazed at how many friends are in the same boat as me. You have a wealth of free exercise buddies waiting for your call. Carve out a convenient but movement oriented activity you can do.

I have a friend who is a 7-minute drive from me, and she has two bicycles. I drive to her, we jump on the bikes and take a 5-mile trip to our favorite organic juice/coffee house, chat business for 30 minutes, then get back on the bikes and drive back. That's 10 total miles of movement that I hardly even feel because I'm so excited to get to the destination.

Keep it simple. Agree on an early morning time frame that not only gets you up and out of bed but gets you back in time to start your day. Most of the time I'm not breaking a sweat so I don't even have to wash my hair. I'm adding this here because I know all the stops and excuses we broads can have. But a one-mile walk around the block with a neighbor twice a week adds up to so much health. Remember, inconsistent is better than never.

Here's a secret for you: I haven't spent that much time in a gym. People think I work out 3-6 days a week. It's because whenever I DO work out I like to post about it on social media. I have been able to inspire thousands of women to add a little extra movement into their life and that makes me so happy! But interestingly enough, when I did the math of all my official workouts in a gym it averages three times a month. Yep, three times a month. Now that is not including washing my car, sweeping my floors, and only taking staircases over elevators. So, from the age of 20-59 years old I have averaged a formal work out three times a month. I'm telling you this because, for me, my "naturally skinny" body has come primarily from food choices.

House cleaning burns a lot of calories. Taking the stairs whenever you see them. Airports and shopping malls, stadiums, parks, office buildings. When you see those flights of stairs and it's 1-3 flights just remind yourself that if you were in a gym you'd push harder on a treadmill for 20 minutes compared to the 4 minutes it will take to climb those stairs…but those stairs add up in your healthy bank account. And they are free. This is where my mother's infamous phrase "Make Use of the Free Facilities" really took off. That's the shift in mindset you need to see. It adds up.

Make a conscious choice as you order that ice cream or go for that third slice of pizza and ask yourself: are you willing to put in some extra movement to balance it out, or would it be easier to just pass on the extra portion and save it for another day, event, or party? That's been a very successful action for me to be able to have treats as I remember the times I've said no, thereby earning me an occasional yes.

When it comes to exercise, I've had my spurts. I did Cross-Fit when I was 49 years old for 9 months, and I LOVED it! But it's been easier for me to choose to eat something healthier and say no to junk foods than to work out at a gym every day.

But hey, if you do both, you probably aren't even reading this book.

CHAPTER TWENTY-FIVE

THE FREE FACILITIES
OF LIFE

It was 1978. We had just moved from Long Island to Los Angeles. I was a kid. My newly-divorced mom and I were driving our mustard-colored Datsun B210 through Griffith Park when she said to me, "Niecey, see those families having a BBQ, and putting balloons on the trees? They really know how to make use of the free facilities."

With my mom, this phrase came to mean more than just using a free park to host a birthday party. It meant taking stairs to get a little exercise instead of the elevator. It meant using the hot car dashboard to warm a ham and cheese sandwich. It also meant getting to a party early to help the hostess and staying late to make new friends.

Basically, squeeze all the goodness you can out of every opportunity you find yourself in. Those are the "free facilities" of life.

There are free exercise moments all around your environment. Start shifting from looking at the doldrum hassle of washing your car to getting free exercise and loads of natural, sun drenched vitamin D. It's going to cost you time and money to drive somewhere to do it. Why not combine all those resources into a metabolic stimulating activity?

Daily Activities:

♦ Wash your car, clean your house.

♦ Walk as much as possible to the store, to your local coffee shop, etc.

♦ Park far away. Walk more.

♦ Help people with lifting items or weight-bearing activities.

♦ My golden rule: ALWAYS TAKE THE STAIRS (even if you're carrying luggage).

When Instagram first launched in 2010 I started posting my healthy food images, fashion and "over 40" fitness hacks. The most popular by far was always the posts about choosing stairs over escalators. I travel a lot, and I get so excited to make use of the free facilities, and a steep set of stairs in a vast airport is the perfect mini workout. What makes it even better is that I'm holding my carry-on which acts as a free weight. None of this is easy to do for me. Especially after hours of flying, but here is my thought process that makes doing these little, quick actions a non-negotiable:

I've just spent 2-6 hours of inactivity sitting on a plane—or I'm about to spend 2-6 hours of inactivity sitting on a plane. So what can I do that won't take up any more of my time or re$ources to counteract that and get me a little more fit?! Walk up the dang stairs!! It's 58 seconds of your life, and you are stretching your hip joints and getting blood flowing throughout those stagnant muscles. And, the visual I have strongest? You are helping to prevent a little cellulite formation above those knees...yeeeech! When you think of it this way, you'll probably start to feel like a lazy person allowing yourself to be moved by heavy electronic equipment. Even walking DOWN the stairs especially after a long flight helps stretch out those hamstrings.

I've had people say to me as I am hustling up the stairs past them, "You're much better than I am." I usually just say—in the hopes of inspiring them: "Ya see, I'm not that motivated, so this is MY version of the gym." I think that if I made a TV commercial about this I might put escalators out of business...

Every flight of steps helps. I have a policy for myself that if I need to go four flights or less, I will ALWAYS walk it. Unless I've done a great workout that day (which is rare), I will always find the stairwell—no matter how sketchy it is. Okay, maybe not at night if I'm alone...

This free exercise also is part of my multi-tasking NY mentality. Do it all, do it now. The fact that I can skip the cab, save 25 dollars, walk to the restaurant, and burn the calories before I even sit down to order is ideal living for me.

I'm really trying to drive this home because conscious movement is getting more vital to do. So many of the activities that used to get us to move our bodies now have apps to do them. Adjusting the temperature in your house can be done with an app. Why go out shopping for things when you can lay on your couch and get it all done? Robot vacuums clean our house!

Even getting ready for the day, driving to meetings, and then parking and going into an office has been replaced by the Zoom meetings--and you don't even have to get dressed from the waist down to attend!

Staying fit isn't always about being comfortable. It can be uncomfortable to move our bodies. And the more often we don't move our bodies, the MORE uncomfortable it feels.

The second I think, "Ugh, it's too far..." Or, "Grrr, that's too heavy." I remind myself— "Bitch, this is your ticket to stronger legs, a healthier heart, and feeling fabulous in your favorite jeans—let's go!"

It's not too hard, it's just a challenge with benefits. Lean into it!

Aside from moving, your muscles need manual help to keep the fascia stimulated—which is why I recommend facial massage to my customers. This process helps create oxygen-rich blood flow and releases toxins in your skin and loosens knots and tension. Of course, I love our Gua Sha Stone, but even doing it with your hands will help.

Gua Sha can gently move lymph fluid toward the lymph nodes, supporting the body's natural detoxification processes. This technique can help reduce puffiness and improve circulation.

Athletes like Tom Brady would get pliability massage stretches often while training in the NFL. He would get them before and after each workout. You may not need to do that exactly, but the idea of moving and then massaging your muscles afterward to keep the blood flowing is a great idea. He's also a HUGE proponent of lots of hydration, which is another reason I'm such a fan!

Bottom line: movement is a critical part of my overall health success—and it's a free facility!

CHAPTER TWENTY-SIX

LONGEVITY FOODS: WISDOM FROM A 110-YEAR-OLD

I was recently captivated by an interview with a remarkable 110-year-old gentleman who shared his nutritional secrets for longevity. As I listened to his clear-minded insights, I couldn't help but be inspired by how vibrant he remained even after eleven decades of life. His voice carried the weight of experience as he outlined his top five recommended foods—simple ingredients that have sustained him through generations of changing dietary trends. Here are the treasures of wisdom he shared:

Raw Honey

Raw honey is full of beneficial enzymes. Use it in tea and coffee for a natural sweetener. Try adding a bit of Himalayan salt to honey before bed—studies show this combination really helps to give you a good night's sleep.

Garlic

Add garlic to your meals by cutting and crushing it in salad dressings and roasted vegetables. Try placing garlic slices on zucchini with Parmesan cheese and roasting them. I sauté vegetables with eggs and garlic regularly. Garlic enhances my Asian salads with sesame and vinegar. Even an avocado becomes more flavorful with a little grated cheese, lemon, and garlic. Try garlic slices with two poached eggs, arugula, feta, and sunflower seed oil for a delicious meal.

Olive Oil

Use olive oil to scramble eggs and enhance soups. Pour it directly into an avocado half with garlic, pistachio nuts, and parmesan for a simple, nutritious treat.

Cinnamon

I now add cinnamon to my coffee whenever it's available. It pairs wonderfully with nut butter and dates.

Chocolate

With chocolate, the darker the better. High-quality dark chocolate provides more health benefits and less sugar than lighter varieties.

CHAPTER TWENTY-SEVEN

MY GROCERY LIST, BROKEN DOWN

Tip: Spend a little more time food shopping. Discover new items especially in the produce section. Also, look at the international section as you'd be surprised at seeing some of your restaurant-favorite foods and condiments that you can make easily at home with far less fats and way more nutrition. Experiment with a bottle of Asian marinade and some thin rice noodles. You can add all your own fresh scallions, slivered carrots, cashews, sliced chicken or scrambled eggs for protein.

We feel we don't have time to cook, but many times we are watching cooking shows while eating the food we had delivered. Spend more time in your own kitchen than watching others. Although, if you are indulging in some TV time, cooking shows can be inspiring and educational.

Nuts

Let's talk about nuts. I'm nuts for nuts. I was a vegetarian on and off for 20 years. I'm not now, but I really got to have quite the love affair with the proteins that you get from nuts. They are my go-to when I need to grab a snack at a gas station. I'm telling you, even if they're roasted and salted and not organic, it's still a healthier deposit into your BBA than a candy bar or bag of chips. If I'm food shopping and I'm starving, I will grab a small bag of nuts right there in the market and eat them while food shopping (saving the bag and paying for it when I check out!) and this is a healthy way to level out my blood sugar and curb over-buying while food shopping because you are starving. This also helps me buy less sweets that I crave when I'm overly hungry and a bit stressed.

Nuts contain monounsaturated and polyunsaturated fats, (NOT trans fats), which help support hormonal balance, reduce inflammation, and improve cardiovascular health. This helps with bone density.

I have a friend in Hollywood who is a casting director and will be at the studio sometimes from 9am till 10pm. She knows her blood sugar drops and will fall prey to the vending machine junk snacks or the late night conference room pizza if she doesn't have her healthy protein snacks throughout the day. She always packs Ziplock bags of nut-filled trail mix, soy nuts, and beef jerky in her purse. And this doesn't mean she has to always say no to the pizza—but maybe having just one slice instead of three—and she was able to resist those vending machine chips.

I started to feel real fancy when I put my nuts in a jar... My husband can't say that sentence. Haha! I love seeing them and not having to roll and clip the bag they were purchased in. It makes me use them more, which is a good thing as they satisfy hunger craving and lower blood sugar levels and can be tossed into oatmeal breakfasts, lunchtime salads and supper stir frys. Glass jars are helpful for oat-meal and quinoa and rice too. Seeing the item does some-thing to your senses and makes you want to use them more. Same thing with fruits and veggies that don't have to be refrigerated-keep them in a bowl on your kitchen counter.

Out of sight out of mind works with our eating habits too.

My Favorite Nuts

Cashews have a lot of copper and manganese which can help protect against heart disease. Cashews, although they taste really fatty, actually have no cholesterol. When you're upping your intake of high density fats, like nuts you're actually helping your liver to clean your body. So cashews, though a little pricey, are very worth it.

Almonds are packed with magnesium, which helps reg-ulate stress hormones, keeping both skin and mood bal-anced. With fiber for digestion, protein for strength, and anti-inflammatory benefits, they're a perfect daily indul-gence for beauty, energy and vitality at any age. Rich in vitamin E, they act as a natural skin shield, fighting free radicals and keeping skin soft, supple, and resilient. Their healthy fats and antioxidants support collagen produc-tion....and who doesn't want more collagen?!

Sunflower seeds are the opposite of pricey and very eas-ily available. Now, raw unsalted are the best for you, but I feel it's an acquired taste and not always easy to find. Sometimes I buy both raw unsalted and roasted salted and mix them together in a jar. Sunflower seeds have a high amount of vitamin E and zinc along with all the other antioxidant and anti-inflammatory properties and are good for hormonal health.

And again, roasted and salted nuts that you pick up at a gas station are still better than that glazed donut or strange chicken sandwich sitting under that hot lamp for hours.

Pumpkin seeds, flax seeds and sesame seeds can increase the overall estrogen in your body. This may relieve some of the symptoms caused by the hormonal depletion during menopause, including hot flashes.

Walnuts are almost considered the king in the nut world. They have a lot of potential for disease-fighting properties and are very high in omega-3 fatty acids which is great for heart health. They also have polyphenols which are antioxidants that help to reduce inflammation.

If you've ever been to Manhattan in the winter you'll see the roasted chestnut carts on the street—THOSE are a healthy single food snack. I went to Istanbul Turkey for a wedding and as I walked the streets, they were filled with roasted chestnuts as a snack for sale. Choose those over the sugar-filled chocolate donuts, soft-serve ice cream or churros.

Now, my favorite nut, being an Italian, is the Mediterranean pistachio nut. Yes, it's very expensive, but being sick is even pricier. Even in my broke college days I knew splurging on healthy snacks in the long-run would keep medical bills down.

I would get really big quantities because if I have a lot I'm going to eat them. Similarly, if you have a lot of potato chips you're going to eat them. So it's a good idea to buy a lot of the things that are healthy for you and find creative ways to add them into your diet.

Nut Butters

Cashew, almond, and sunflower seed butters are a glow-up from peanut butter, offering better nutrition and skin benefits. Peanut butter's high omega-6s and potential mold (aflatoxins) can trigger inflammation, while these alternatives are rich in vitamin E, zinc, and magnesium—essential for collagen, hydration, and stress balance. Plus, they're gentler on digestion and packed with skin-loving antioxidants.

You can do so much with nut butters: A sunflower seed butter and honey sandwich on Ezekiel toast…Yum! Almond butter in a vanilla protein powder oat milk cacao smoothie. Any nut butter (even peanut without added sugars) and celery is a nutritious hunger satisfier.

Nuts are like your body's tiny personal trainers—boosting the good cholesterol (HDL) while keeping the bad in check. Packed with healthy fats, fiber, and protein, they keep you full, curb cravings, and rev up metabolism. Despite their calorie count, they actually help burn fat, not store it. So go ahead, grab a handful—your heart and waistline will thank you!

Quinoa

Let's talk about *quinoa*—this tiny, mighty powerhouse that's been around for thousands of years, but it still feels like a secret weapon for vibrant health! I mean, it's a complete protein. Yes, *complete*! That means it's got all nine essential amino acids your body needs—without you having to pair it with anything else. That's time-saving meal prep right there!

Another benefit is that it's not actually a grain! It's a *seed*—which means it's naturally gluten-free and easier to digest for a lot of people.

It's packed with nutrients. Magnesium, iron, B vitamins, fiber... basically, your skin, your digestion, your energy levels? They all *love* quinoa. It's like feeding your body *real* fuel, not just filler carbs. So if you've ever felt *meh* after eating traditional grains, quinoa might just be your new best friend.

My husband is celiac and can't have gluten. When my daughter was born in 1994 quinoa wasn't very popular but I knew about it as a safer grain and when I noticed some diaper and facial rashes as a toddler, I swapped out regular semolina wheat flour pasta with quinoa. I made it in a rice cooker and added tomato sauce and parmesan cheese, or melted cheddar cheese for a protein rich healthy mac & cheese. I also love to add chicken or vegetable bouillon and sauté the cooked quinoa with mushrooms and fresh garlic.

You can make a glow-boosting quinoa salad and add roasted sweet potatoes, avocado, arugula garbanzos and lemon tahini dressing (liquid gold!).

Cheese

Cheese is an Italian staple, but not as popular in Asian culture which was the other half of my cooking inspiration growing up. I learned early on that there are qualities of cheese and it should only be a small part of a dish, not the main meal—even though my "last meal" would probably be baked macaroni and cheese and garlic mashed potatoes, smothered in butter and salt. But, I digress... And, while I'm alive and thriving I try whenever possible to stay away from processed cheese food (like nachos from a snack bar or restaurant) and choose cheeses easier to digest.

Aged hard cheeses such as parmesan, goat cheese, and cheddar have less lactose, meaning fewer side effects for the lactose-intolerant.

Here are some hard aged cheeses that are low in lactose: Parmesan, Cheddar, Swiss, Colby & Monterey Jack.

Below are other notable healthier cheese options.

Goat cheese is easier to digest than cow's milk cheese because it has different proteins and it has medium-chain fatty acids that the body absorbs quickly.

Cottage cheese is low in fat and carbohydrates. As protein comprises more than two thirds of the calories in cottage cheese, it's a good food to eat before or after exercise or simply when you want to stay feeling fuller for longer.

Feta cheese is practically lactose-free, and is lower in fat than many cheeses. It's a good source of vitamins and minerals, including phosphorus, and selenium.

Soft fresh mozzarella is lower in sodium and calories than most other cheeses. It contains probiotics that may benefit your immune system.

Blue and Brie cheeses are good for those who are lactose-intolerant because of how they are aged. The aging process breaks down lactose.

Avoid processed cheeses like American and deli Swiss—they're made by melting natural cheese with whey and other additives, such as emulsifying salts, vegetable oils, butterfat, and other dairy ingredients.

Also stay away from bright orange liquid and canned cheeses, as they will absolutely age you. Ironically, the aged cheeses do not age you!

You don't need to eat reduced-fat cheese because they usually are adding some filler ingredients that are not as digestible to your body and can be worse for your health than the fat that it's trying to replace.

Just writing this I can feel the belly fat forming!

Beans

Now… beans! Beans are soluble fibers, which means they absorb like a sponge. Our liver is our main detoxification organ. Along with the pancreas and gallbladder, it acts as a filter for our gastrointestinal tract. The liver produces bile, which, like dish soap, breaks up the fats and frees up compounds to be digested and filtered. That bile goes from the liver to the intestine and back again as a cycle. But who cleans out the bile before it returns to your liver?

Beans! Soluble fibers bind to the toxins to help escort them OUT of your body. Psyllium husks will do the same thing too. Regular elimination is vital to prevent a sluggish, tired body, poor sleep, brain fog, and acne breakouts. It's like a trash can that never gets emptied. So add that cup of garbanzo or kidney beans to your salad.

I will eat an entire can of garbanzo for lunch. Now, I know that might sound extreme, but I've heard of people eating an entire pint of ice cream in one sitting or two, or Chips Ahoy! cookies, or an entire large bag of Doritos. And yet, eating a whole can of one of the healthiest foods for our bodies has sometimes been met with shock.

Garbanzos to me, are like dairy-free chunks of cheese— they are like the soft croutons of the bean world. They fill me with protein, nutrients, and make me feel like I'm eating some kind of bad-for-me comfort food. If you like garbanzo beans then you understand what I'm talking about. If you don't, well, there are other healthy protein snacks…

Lentil soup is another great source of protein, and it's usually not made with fatty meats or cheeses, making it a smart choice at a restaurant. If you buy it in a can, use my healthy tip which I mentioned earlier: add fresh vegetables to the soup base and raise the deposit to your BBA.

Also, if you find yourself at a fast food Mexican restaurant, it's always the lesser of evils to get a side of black beans, a side salad, and many times they can give you just a side of grilled chicken. You don't have to be totally anti-social and never get anything on the menu, but it's good to know which foods are the least harmful, and that you can always ask for a stripped-down version of something without toxic liquid cheese and questionable fatty meat.

With my daughter, from about the age of four until she was a teenager, I would give her a little snack bowl in her room while she played or watched a movie. It usually had tomatoes, baby carrots, and a handful of either red kidney beans or garbanzo beans. And she would always finish it all.

One night we were having dinner and a friend of mine was with us and she said to my daughter "you hardly ate any of your pasta," and I told my friend, "It's totally fine, she had her veggies and protein about an hour ago. So it's okay if she doesn't finish that bowl of yummy starch."

I lived on bean burritos most of my younger years. I was a not-so-strict vegetarian, so bean, cheese and veggie bur- ritos were a staple for me. I primarily made them at home because I knew I was getting cleaner beans. Refried beans at restaurants are filled with lard and should be eaten spar- ingly. But you are able to get canned refried beans that are less fatty. And whenever you can do whole black or pinto beans where you know they haven't added additional fats and oils which ultimately make it deliciously but unhealth- ily creamy, you're doing a better deposit to your BBA.

P.S. Any discomfort you might get adding beans to your diet will lessen with time as your body adjusts to this healthy habit.

Wilted Vegetables

We've all had vegetables wilt right before our eyes in our fridges, and a little discolored. When I was in college I couldn't afford to buy a lot of vegetables, and nowadays organic vegetables are very expensive, so I just squeeze the usage out of them to the last minute. The internet says it doesn't make them inedible. All right, it may change the flavor a tad but that's what you know onions and garlic are for. You could sauté them up with eggs, you can make soups or stews.

It's really just a matter of viewpoint shift because you know someone will have non-dairy creamer which is complete belly-fat-producing, or diet soda which is totally toxic and ruins your adrenals. So, a deflated piece of kale is way more your body's friend than hydrogenated oil and Nu-traSweet.

Fermented Food

Fermented foods have been healing humans for centuries. They are a vital part of many cultures and are made through an ancient process that involves using live micro-organisms to preserve food and add nutritional value.

Kombucha drinks actually come from black tea. It's primarily just plain brewed tea with sugar and a piece of fermented bacteria called a SCOBY. Like when you make kefir you have what's called "kefir grains" which are live bacteria that infuse probiotics into the milk.

Yogurt is made in a similar fashion by using yogurt starter (what came first, the yogurt or the starter?… Okay, I thought that was funny). And then there is a fermented starter you need to make any sourdough bread. It's actually why sourdough is a healthier gut choice when it comes to choosing bread because the fermentation process creates prebiotics, which feed the beneficial bacteria in your gut and helps to break down the carbohydrates. It potentially aids digestion and promotes a healthy microbiome—this is especially true when choosing whole wheat sourdough for added fiber content.

Fermented foods like kimchi, tempeh, miso soup and apple cider vinegar also make healthy additions to your BBA.

Sauerkraut and pickles are common examples of fermented foods. So if you're at the baseball game and you have to eat that nitrate filled hotdog (preferably without the bun) add sauerkraut and pickles to give your gut a little deposit into your BBA to make up for the withdrawal that the hot dog is taking out of it. Oh, and use mustard instead of ketchup whenever possible—mustard has no sugar and fewer calories. Or at the very least, just use less ketchup.

Nourish your gut and it'll return the favor with a radiant glow, boundless energy and balanced hormones. Fermented foods are nature's alchemy—alive with probiotics. Your skin and body will thank you for giving it that lit-from-within magic.

Bell Pepper

I used to not be a fan of them. Now I can't get enough of them, especially the orange and yellow and the red. Did you know that they have twice as many grams of Vitamin

C than an orange? They have half the carbs, half the sugar, and they make a really satisfying, crunchy snack—perfect when you're craving that crunch but want something better than a cracker, cookie, or chip to sink your teeth into. They're kind of awesome because all you have to do when you're sitting at your desk and you just want to eat a junky snack, is you can grab one of these babies and chomp it whole. I eat it like an apple.

They're savory and a tad sweet. There's so much flavor to it that you feel satisfied. It doesn't have the sugars or carbohydrates of most fruits, and they have 190 mg of Vitamin C, and an orange has just 69 mg. Crazy right?! And of course Vitamin C is great for collagen, which is great for your joints, and… your lovely face!

FOODIE FLASHCARDS

1. Share calories. Always offer others some of whatever you're eating.
2. Eat less sugar. This also means choosing savory over sweet.
3. Don't eat by the clock.
4. Don't eat if you're not hungry.
5. Hydrate. Drink electrolyte water and tea.
6. Avoid alcohol. It's dehydrating.
7. Buy your produce fresh from the market over frozen/canned.
8. Focus on foods with less ingredients, read the labels.

9. Small plates and bowls equals small portions, *except* for large salad bowls.

10. Buy less pre-cooked, packaged meals.

SNACKS

- Crispy cinnamon apple chips
- Hard boiled eggs
- Cottage cheese
- Hummus
- Nitrate-free, non-GMO beef/turkey sticks
- Apple sauce (no sugar added)
- Walnuts
- Fruit leather
- Sweet and savory rice cakes
- Seaweed snacks
- Celery and nut butter
- Cucumber and tzatziki sauce/tahini sauce
- Trail mix
- Pumpkin seeds
- Pistachio nuts (in shell to slow eating speed)
- Raw bell peppers
- Cucumbers
- Sliced radishes soaked in Bragg's liquid aminos, sesame seed oil, and a splash of rice vinegar (apple cider vinegar is okay too!)

FOODS THAT SUPPORT RADIANT, HEALTHY SKIN

Eat More Of These:

- Broccoli
- Sweet potatoes
- Avocados
- Grass-fed butter
- Cauliflower
- Beets

- Asparagus
- Olives
- Pumpkin
- Kale
- Brussels sprouts
- Romaine lettuce
- Cucumbers
- Salmon (wild-caught)
- Eggs (pasture-raised)
- Papaya
- Blueberries
- Tomatoes
- Walnuts/pecans
- Spinach
- Red/orange bell peppers
- Turmeric
- Bone broth
- Chia seeds
- Lemons
- Green tea
- Fresh raw Garlic and Onion
- Olive Oil

FOODS, INGREDIENTS, AND HABITS TO AVOID FOR HEALTHY SKIN

Cut Back or Eliminate:

Food & Beverage:

- Alcohol (wine and cocktail–big dehydrators and inflammation)
- Refined sugar
- Processed foods (so many packaged meals and pastries)
- Excessive refined Grains (white flour-white rice)
- Soda
- Dairy (especially conventional)
- High-glycemic carbs (white bread, white rice, pastries)
- Artificial sweeteners (aspartame, sucralose)

- MSG (monosodium glutamate ask if your chinese take-out has it)
- Vegetable oils (canola, corn)

- Nitrates/nitrites (processed meats bacon [i know!], many deli meats)
- Excess caffeine
- Food dyes (Red 40, Yellow 5, etc.)

Lifestyle & Topicals:

- Cigarettes
- Cheap synthetic-filled skincare products
- Parabens
- Stearates

- Sodium lauryl sulfate (SLS)
- Synthetic fragrance/ parfum

Want to glow from the inside out? Stick with whole, colorful, anti-inflammatory foods, and be just as picky about what goes on your skin as what goes in your body!

MY SHOPPING LIST:

Eggs/Dairy

- Eggs
- Raw cheese whenever possible.
- Parmesan cheese

- Feta cheese
- Cottage Cheese
- Irish butter

Add-ons

- Olive oil
- Flax seeds

- Spirulina powder

- Wheat grass juice powder (although fresh shots are great!)
- Vegetable bouillon cubes
- Apple cider vinegar
- Rice vinegar
- Mayonnaise (with the least ingredients)
- MCT oil
- Sesame seed oil
- Bragg's aminos (Tastes like soy sauce!)

Grains

- Ezekiel bread
- Quinoa (which is actually a seed not a grain)
- Scandinavian crackers
- Muesli cereal

Nuts & Beans

- Almonds
- Walnuts
- Pistachios (with shell-takes longer to eat)
- Sunflower seeds
- Toasted pumpkin seeds
- Canned garbanzo beans
- Humus

Vegetables

- Red, orange, yellow bell peppers
- Radishes
- Fresh Kale
- Green beans
- Chives
- Green onions
- Asparagus
- Basil leaves
- Carrots
- Celery
- Radishes
- Bok choy
- Beets with green leaves
- Cucumber (small Persian style)

- Onions
- Garlic
- Zucchini

- Ginger
- Turmeric

Fruit

- Pineapple
- Clementines (cuties)
- Banana

- Lemons & lemon juice in a small bottle
- Jelly preserves without sugar
- Frozen berries

Meat (try to get organic & hormone-free)

- Tuna fish in water
- Salmon
- Chicken

- Steak
- Chop meat

Drinks

- Coconut water
- Green tea hot or cold
- Chai tea
- Club soda (with lemon juice and a drop of monk fruit or stevia sweetener)

- Water with ginger turmeric, apple cider vinegar
- Kombucha

- Almond or coconut milk unsweetened

A Meal Plan Idea From This Shopping List:

Breakfast

2 eggs, one slice Ezekiel bread with Irish butter

or

Protein smoothie made from whatever I have: Nut milk, flax seeds, spirulina, raw egg, protein powder, collagen, MCT oil, frozen blueberries, half a frozen banana, instant coffee, powdered amino acids

Snack

Clementines, bell peppers, pistachios, beef or turkey stick

Lunch

Tuna fish with lots of finely chopped celery and any kind of onion for fiber (chives, scallions, red onion) a tablespoon of mayonnaise, lemon juice salt and pepper

Scandinavian crackers – just 2

or

1 cup Cottage cheese, 2 crackers, chopped salad of raw veggies

or

Quinoa sautéed with pieces of chicken, (chives or green onion) sesame seed oil, Bragg's amino & raw celery and carrot sticks

Dinner

Steam-sautéed zucchini with chicken, quinoa with a vegetable broth cube or better than bouillon, olive oil and or butter and a teeny bit of shaved parmesan

or

Chopped salad of massaged kale, micro-greens, chopped cucumber, tomatoes, bell peppers, sunflower seeds, pistachios and feta cheese

RECIPE APPENDIX

Cooking, to me, is part intuition, part mood, and part "what's-about-to-go-bad-in-the-fridge." That said, I've jotted down a few structured recipes for those who like a game plan. Feel free to treat them as suggestions, not commandments. Use them as a base, then freestyle your way to something uniquely yours.

Salad Dressings

Feel free to vary ingredients based on what you have in your kitchen!

French Dijon: 1 Tbsp Red wine, 1 tsp dijon mustard, 1 clove garlic, ½ tsp oregano, 3 Tbsp olive oil, salt and pepper to taste

Creamy French: ¼ c.Greek yogurt, 1 Tbsp olive oil, 1 Tbsp lemon juice, 1 clove minced garlic clove, 1 tsp Dijon mustard, salt and pepper to taste

Mediterranean Vinaigrette: 2 Tbsp Lemon juice, 1 Tbsp Apple cider vinegar, 2 Tbsp olive oil, 1 tsp finely chopped onion or shallots & garlic, ½ tsp dried oregano

Avocado Dressing: 1 large avocado, 1/4 small yellow onion finely chopped, 2-3 scallions, 2 clove garlic, ¼ c fresh parsley, ½ fresh basil leaves, ¼ c olive oil, 3 Tbsp lemon juice, 3 Tbsp ACV, salt and pepper, food processor or blender

Creamy Asian Dressing: 1 Tbsp toasted sesame seeds, ¼ cup Sesame seed oil, 3 Tbsp mayo, ¼ cup low sodium soy sauce, 1 tsp brown sugar, 1 Tbsp olive oil, 1 tsp rice wine vinegar

Asian-Carrot Dressing: ¾ cup olive oil, ¼ cup sesame seed oil, ⅓ cup rice wine vinegar, 2 carrots roughly chopped, 4 green onions (white part only) sliced, 1 clove garlic, 2 Tbsp minced ginger, 2 Tbsp low sodium soy sauce, 1 Tbsp honey, blend in blender

Soups and Salads

Salad Puree Soup

So, you've got a fridge full of **sad, wilted** veggies that have seen better days? How about all that leftover salad that's giving you the side-eye? Fear not, those "expired" (but not moldy!) vegetables are just waiting for their second chance at greatness—**in a soup puree!**

The Golden Rules of Soup Alchemy:

1. "Limp" Does Not Mean "Lifeless"

Just because your spinach looks like it just pulled an all-nighter doesn't mean it's useless. They are packed with flavor and when you lightly cook them, they are easier on your digestion and still full of nutrition. So those wilted greens, bendy carrots, and even that slightly squishy zucchini are **perfect for soup.**

We're going to blend them into a no-waste, homemade creamy soup. The pureed texture makes any imperfections or signs of aging unnoticeable. It cooks in 30 minutes and you only need one pot and it is very low calorie.

2. Sniff Before You Simmer

If it's moldy, slimy, or smells funny, toss it. If it just looks tired but smells fine—game on!

3. Roast for Flavor Boost

If you feel up to it, roast your veggies on a baking sheet with a little oil, salt, and garlic, at 400°F for 20-30 min. This caramelizes them, bringing out hidden flavors!

4. The Big Blend-Up

- Sauté an onion and some garlic in a pot (always the base of greatness).
- Add your veggies or salad and some broth or water (about 4 cups).
- Simmer for 20 minutes.
- BLEND! Use an immersion blender or a regular blender (careful, it's hot!).

Look, I go a bit rogue when it comes to strict recipes—I'll dance around it and see where the flavor takes me. After all, some of the best dishes I've made happen when I follow my instincts in the kitchen. But my editor insists that I give you something a little more structured. So here are some recipes you can follow as a roadmap of healthy dishes… Though I fully support a little detour if inspiration strikes!

Salad Soup Puree

Ingredients:

- 2 cups leftover salad— dressed or undressed (ex; arugula, romaine, spinach, kale, cucumbers, tomatoes, beans, onions)
- 1 tbsp vinaigrette

For the soup:

- 1 tsp olive oil
- 300 ml vegetable stock (or from cube)

Instructions:

1. Heat the olive oil in a saucepan, and add the salad.
2. Fry for a few minutes.
3. Add the stock, put on the lid and simmer for about 10 minutes.
4. Blend until smooth.
5. Season to taste with salt and pepper.

Rustic Root Puree

Ingredients:

- Salt, pepper and garlic powder to taste
- 2 medium potatoes (russet and/or sweet potatoes)
- 1/2 head of cauliflower and broccoli
- 6 Carrots or 2 cups of baby carrots
- A can of corn or 3/4 bag of frozen corn
- Veggie bouillon cube or paste

Instructions:

1. Dice all the veggies.
2. Add them to a large pot.
3. Cover with water and bring to boil then simmer for 20 minutes.
4. Add the corn in the last 10 minutes.
5. Drain water and set water aside.
6. Puree the veggies with an immersion blender.
7. Add vegetable bouillon to the water and add about a cup or so of that seasoned water back until you get the desired soup texture.

Nitrate-free Antipasto-Style Salad

Ingredients:

- **For the Salad:**

- 1/2 head iceberg lettuce or 2 small romaine hearts, sliced into strips
- 1 head radicchio, sliced into strips
- 1/2 medium red onion, thinly sliced
- 1 pint cherry tomatoes, quartered

- 1 can chickpeas, rinsed and drained
- 5 pepperoncini, stemmed and sliced
- 3/4 cup cubed mozzarella cheese
- Sea salt and freshly ground black pepper, to taste

- **For the Dressing:**

- 1/3 cup extra-virgin olive oil
- 2-3 tablespoons lemon juice (or juice from one squeezed lemon)
- 2 tablespoons red wine vinegar
- 1/2 shallot, finely chopped

- 2 garlic cloves, finely chopped
- 1 tablespoon dried oregano
- 1/2 teaspoon sea salt
- Freshly ground black pepper to taste

Instructions:

1. **Prepare the Dressing:**

- In a small bowl, whisk together the olive oil, lemon juice, red wine vinegar, finely chopped shallot, garlic, dried oregano, 1/2 teaspoon of sea salt, and freshly ground black pepper until well combined. Set aside.

2. **Prepare the Salad:**

♦ Slice the iceberg lettuce or romaine hearts and radicchio into lengthwise strips.

♦ In a large bowl, combine the sliced lettuce, radicchio, thinly sliced red onion, quartered cherry tomatoes, chickpeas, mozzarella cubes, and sliced pepperoncini.

3. **Dress the Salad:**

♦ Drizzle the prepared dressing over the salad ingredients.

♦ Toss the salad gently to coat all the ingredients evenly with the dressing.

♦ Season with additional salt and pepper, if desired, and toss again.

4. **Serve:**

♦ Sprinkle with extra dried oregano, if desired, and serve immediately.

Enjoy your refreshing and crunchy antipasto-style salad!

Simple Arugula Salad with Salmon

Salad Ingredients:

- 4 cups arugula
- 1/4 cup shaved Parmesan cheese
- 1/4 cup pistachios, sunflower seeds, cashews, or roasted chickpeas (choose your favorite)
- 1/2 red onion, thinly sliced

Dressing Ingredients:

- 1/4 cup olive oil
- 2 tablespoons apple cider vinegar
- A splash of balsamic vinegar
- 1 teaspoon Dijon mustard
- 1 garlic clove, finely chopped

Salmon:

- 2 salmon fillets
- 1 tablespoon olive oil
- 2-3 tablespoons water
- Salt and pepper, to taste

Instructions:

1. **Prepare the Dressing:**

- In a small bowl, whisk together olive oil, apple cider vinegar, balsamic vinegar, Dijon mustard, and finely chopped garlic. Set aside.

2. **Prepare the Salad:**

- In a large salad bowl, combine arugula, shaved Parmesan cheese, your choice of nuts or roasted chickpeas, and thinly sliced red onion.

3. **Cook the Salmon:**

- Heat olive oil in a skillet over medium-high heat.
- Place the salmon fillets in the skillet, skin side down.
- Add 2-3 tablespoons of water to the skillet.
- Cover the skillet with a lid and allow the salmon to steam and sear for about 5-7 minutes, or until the salmon is cooked through and flakes easily with a fork.
- Season with salt and pepper to taste. Remove from heat and let it rest for a minute.

4. **Assemble the Salad:**

- Drizzle the dressing over the arugula salad and toss gently to coat the ingredients evenly.
- Divide the salad onto plates and top each with a salmon fillet.

5. **Serve:**

- Serve the salad with salmon immediately, enjoying the combination of flavors and textures.

Enjoy your healthy and delicious arugula salad with salmon!

Asian Cucumber Salad

Ingredients:

- 4 Persian cucumbers, thinly sliced into circles (or 1 regular cucumber)
- 3-4 radishes, thinly sliced
- 1 tablespoon chopped onion
- 1/2 cup apple cider vinegar
- 1/2 cup rice vinegar (or substitute with red wine vinegar or white vinegar with a pinch of sugar)
- 2 tablespoons sesame oil
- 2 tablespoons Bragg's amino acids or soy sauce
- Onion powder, to taste
- Garlic powder, to taste

Instructions:

1. **Prepare the Vegetables:**
   - Thinly slice the cucumbers and radishes. Chop the onion.

2. **Combine Ingredients:**
   - Place the sliced cucumbers, radishes, and chopped onion in a large bowl or Tupperware.

3. **Make the Dressing:**
   - In a separate bowl, whisk together apple cider vinegar, rice vinegar, sesame oil, and Bragg's amino acids or soy sauce.

4. **Mix the Salad:**
   - Pour the dressing over the vegetables in the bowl.
   - Add onion powder and garlic powder to taste.

5. **Chill and Serve:**
   - Mix all the ingredients until well combined.

- Let the salad sit for a minimum of 15 minutes before serving to enhance the flavors.
- Store the salad in the refrigerator. The flavors will continue to develop and improve overnight.

Enjoy this refreshing, gut healthy and flavorful Asian cucumber salad!

My Grandmas Chicken Veggie Salad

Ingredients:

- 2 carrots, chopped
- 2 celery stalks, chopped
- 1/2 cup onion, chopped
- 1 can chopped chicken, drained
- 1/3 cup raisins and/or 1/2 cup apple, chopped
- 1/2 cup walnuts
- 3 tablespoons mayonnaise or vegenaise
- 3 tablespoons apple cider vinegar
- Pinch of onion powder
- Celtic or himalayan salt

Instructions:

1. **Prepare the Ingredients:**

- Chop the carrots, celery, onion, and apple (if using).
- Drain the canned chicken.

2. **Combine Ingredients:**

- In a large bowl, combine the chopped carrots, celery, onion, and canned chicken.
- Add the raisins and/or chopped apple and walnuts to the bowl.

3. **Make the Dressing:**

- In a separate small bowl, mix the mayonnaise (or vegenaise) with the apple cider vinegar and onion powder.

4. **Assemble the Salad:**

- Pour the dressing over the salad ingredients in the large bowl.
- Toss everything together until all the ingredients are well coated with the dressing.

5. **Chill and Serve:**

♦ For best flavor, let the salad sit in the refrigerator for at least 30 minutes before serving.

♦ Serve the salad cold as a refreshing and nutritious meal.

Kale/Arugula Egg Salad

Ingredients:

- 1-2 handfuls of kale or arugula (or both)
- 1 tablespoon butter
- 1 egg
- 1 teaspoon apple cider vinegar (ACV) or balsamic vinegar
- 1/4 cup small tomatoes, chopped
- Pinch of black pepper
- 1 garlic clove, minced (or garlic powder to taste)
- 1 tablespoon water
- Shaved Parmesan cheese

Instructions:

1. **Prepare the Greens:**

- Chop the kale then massage in a bowl with olive oil and salt to get the bitter taste out and then arrange on a plate.

2. **Cook the Egg:**

- Melt the butter in a coated pan over medium heat.
- Crack the egg into the pan and let it cook for about 20 seconds.
- Add one tablespoon of water to the pan and cover it with a lid to steam/poach the egg without flipping.
- Cook until the egg white is set but the yolk is still runny.

3. **Assemble the Salad:**

- Slide the cooked egg on top of the kale/arugula.
- Drizzle with a teaspoon of apple cider vinegar or balsamic vinegar.
- Add the chopped tomatoes over the greens.

4. **Season the Salad:**

♦ Sprinkle with a pinch of black pepper and add minced garlic or garlic powder to taste.

♦ Top with shaved Parmesan cheese.

5. **Serve:**

♦ Serve the salad immediately for a fresh and flavorful meal.

Bean Salad

Ingredients:

- 1 can garbanzo beans, drained
- 1 can kidney beans, drained
- 1 cup cherry tomatoes, sliced in half
- 1/2 red onion, thinly sliced

Dressing:

- 1/4 cup olive oil
- 2 cloves garlic, chopped
- 2 tablespoons balsamic vinegar

Instructions:

1. **Prepare the Ingredients:**
- Drain the garbanzo beans and kidney beans.
- Slice the cherry tomatoes in half and thinly slice the red onion.

2. **Make the Dressing:**
- In a small bowl, whisk together the olive oil, chopped garlic, and balsamic vinegar until well combined.

3. **Assemble the Salad:**
- In a large bowl, combine the garbanzo beans, kidney beans, cherry tomatoes, and sliced red onion.

4. **Dress the Salad:**
- Pour the dressing over the salad ingredients.
- Toss gently to ensure all the ingredients are evenly coated with the dressing.

5. **Serve:**

♦ Serve the salad immediately, or let it sit for 15 minutes to allow the flavors to meld.

Enjoy your refreshing and nutritious bean salad!

Italian-Style Curried Cauliflower Soup

Ingredients:

- 1 large head of cauliflower, cut into florets
- 1 tablespoon olive oil
- 1 medium onion, chopped
- 2 cloves garlic, minced
- 1 tablespoon curry powder
- 1 teaspoon dried oregano
- 1/2 teaspoon dried basil
- 1/4 teaspoon red pepper flakes (optional)
- 4 cups chicken or vegetable broth
- 1 cup canned coconut milk (full-fat for creaminess)
- 1/2 cup grated Parmesan cheese
- Salt and black pepper, to taste
- Fresh basil or parsley, chopped (for garnish)

Instructions:

1. **Prepare the Cauliflower:**
- Cut the cauliflower into florets.

2. **Sauté the Aromatics:**
- Heat olive oil in a large pot over medium heat.
- Add the chopped onion and cook for 5-7 minutes, until softened and translucent.
- Stir in the minced garlic and cook for an additional 1-2 minutes, until fragrant.

3. **Add Spices:**
- Add the curry powder, dried oregano, dried basil, and red pepper flakes (if using) to the pot.
- Stir well to coat the onions and garlic with the spices and cook for 1 minute.

4. **Cook the Cauliflower:**

- Add the cauliflower florets to the pot and stir to combine with the spices.
- Pour in the chicken or vegetable broth and bring to a boil.
- Reduce the heat to a simmer and cook for 15-20 minutes, or until the cauliflower is tender.

5. **Blend the Soup:**

- Use an immersion blender to blend the soup until smooth. Alternatively, carefully transfer the soup in batches to a countertop blender and blend until smooth.

6. **Add Coconut Milk:**

- Return the blended soup to the pot if needed.
- Stir in the coconut milk and heat gently until warmed through.
- If using, add the grated Parmesan cheese and stir until melted and well combined.

7. **Season and Serve:**

- Season with salt and black pepper to taste.
- Garnish with freshly chopped basil or parsley.

Enjoy your creamy and flavorful Italian-style curried Paleo cauliflower soup!

Vegetables

Sautéed Broccoli

Ingredients:

- 1 large head of broccoli (about 4 cups florets)
- 2 tablespoons olive oil
- 2 cloves garlic, minced
- 1/4 teaspoon red pepper flakes (optional)
- Salt and black pepper, to taste
- 1 tablespoon lemon juice (optional)
- 1/4 cup grated Parmesan cheese (optional)

Instructions:

1. **Prepare the Broccoli:**

- Cut the broccoli into bite-sized florets. If you like, you can also peel and slice the stems into smaller pieces for added texture.

2. **Heat the Oil:**

- In a large skillet, heat the olive oil over medium heat.

3. **Sauté the Broccoli:**

- Add the broccoli florets to the skillet and cook for 5-7 minutes, stirring occasionally, until the broccoli is tender and slightly crispy on the edges.

4. **Add Garlic and Seasonings:**

- Add the minced garlic and red pepper flakes (if using) to the skillet.

- Cook for an additional 1-2 minutes until the garlic is fragrant and lightly golden. Be careful not to burn the garlic.

5. **Season:**

- Season with salt and black pepper to taste.
- If desired, drizzle with lemon juice for extra flavor and freshness.

6. **Optional Garnish:**

- Sprinkle with grated Parmesan cheese before serving, if desired.

7. **Serve:**

- Transfer the sautéed broccoli to a serving dish and enjoy immediately.

This simple and flavorful sautéed broccoli makes a perfect side dish for any meal!

Steamed Mashed Cauliflower

Ingredients:

- 1 large head of cauliflower, cut into florets
- 2 tablespoons olive oil
- 2 cloves garlic, minced
- 1/4 cup milk or non-dairy milk (adjust as needed)
- 1/4 cup grated Parmesan cheese (optional)
- Salt and black pepper, to taste
- Fresh chives or parsley, chopped (optional, for garnish)

Instructions:

1. **Steam the Cauliflower:**

- Place the cauliflower florets in a steamer basket over a pot of simmering water.
- Cover and steam for about 10-12 minutes, or until the cauliflower is very tender when pierced with a fork.

2. **Prepare the Garlic:**

- While the cauliflower is steaming, heat olive oil in a small skillet over medium heat.
- Add the minced garlic and cook for 1-2 minutes, or until fragrant and lightly golden. Be careful not to burn the garlic.

3. **Mash the Cauliflower:**

- Once the cauliflower is tender, transfer it to a large bowl.
- Use a potato masher, fork, or an immersion blender to mash the cauliflower until smooth. For a smoother texture, you can also use a food processor or blender.

4. **Add Flavors:**

* Stir in the cooked garlic and olive oil.

* Gradually add the milk or non-dairy milk until you reach your desired consistency. You can adjust the amount of milk based on how creamy you want the mashed cauliflower to be.

* If using, mix in the grated Parmesan cheese.

* Season with salt and black pepper to taste.

5. **Serve:**

* Transfer the mashed cauliflower to a serving dish.

* Garnish with chopped fresh chives or parsley, if desired.

Enjoy your creamy and flavorful steamed mashed cauliflower as a healthy alternative to mashed potatoes!

Cauliflower Rice

Ingredients:

- 1 large head of cauliflower, cut into florets
- 1 tablespoon coconut oil
- 1 small onion, finely chopped
- 2 cloves garlic, minced
- Salt and black pepper, to taste
- 1/4 cup chopped fresh parsley or cilantro (optional, for garnish)
- 1/2 lemon, juiced (optional, for extra flavor)

Instructions:

1. **Prepare the Cauliflower:**

- Cut the cauliflower into florets.
- Place the florets in a food processor and pulse until the cauliflower resembles rice grains. Do this in batches if necessary to avoid overcrowding the processor.

2. **Cook the Aromatics:**

- Heat coconut oil in a large skillet over medium heat.
- Add the chopped onion and cook for 5-7 minutes, until softened and translucent.
- Stir in the minced garlic and cook for an additional 1 minute, until fragrant.

3. **Cook the Cauliflower Rice:**

- Add the processed cauliflower rice to the skillet with the onions and garlic.
- Cook for 5-7 minutes, stirring occasionally, until the cauliflower is tender and slightly golden. Adjust the

cooking time for your preferred texture—shorter for more al dente, longer for softer rice.

4. **Season and Finish:**

* Season with salt and black pepper to taste.

* If desired, stir in freshly chopped parsley or cilantro for added freshness and flavor.

* For a bright touch, drizzle with a squeeze of lemon juice before serving.

5. **Serve:**

* Transfer the cauliflower rice to a serving dish and enjoy as a healthy alternative to traditional rice.

This cauliflower rice is versatile and can be used as a base for many dishes or served as a side!

Balsamic Roasted Cauliflower

Ingredients:

- 1 large head of cauliflower, cut into florets
- 2 tablespoons extra-virgin olive oil
- 3 tablespoons balsamic vinegar
- 2 tablespoons honey or maple syrup (for a vegan option)
- 1 teaspoon dried thyme
- 1/2 teaspoon garlic powder
- 1/2 teaspoon onion powder
- Salt and black pepper, to taste
- 1/4 cup grated Parmesan cheese (optional, for a non-vegan option)
- Fresh parsley, chopped (for garnish)

Instructions:

1. **Preheat the Oven:**

- Preheat your oven to 425°F (220°C).

2. **Prepare the Cauliflower:**

- Cut the cauliflower into bite-sized florets and place them in a large mixing bowl.

3. **Make the Balsamic Glaze:**

- In a small bowl, whisk together the olive oil, balsamic vinegar, and honey or maple syrup.

4. **Season the Cauliflower:**

- Pour the balsamic mixture over the cauliflower florets.
- Add dried thyme, garlic powder, onion powder, salt, and black pepper.

- Toss the cauliflower until evenly coated with the mixture.

5. **Roast the Cauliflower:**

- Spread the seasoned cauliflower in a single layer on a baking sheet lined with parchment paper or lightly greased.

- Roast in the preheated oven for 20-25 minutes, or until the cauliflower is tender and edges are golden brown. Stir halfway through cooking for even roasting.

6. **Add Parmesan (Optional):**

- If using, sprinkle the grated Parmesan cheese over the cauliflower during the last 5 minutes of roasting, allowing it to melt and lightly brown.

7. **Garnish and Serve:**

- Remove from the oven and garnish with freshly chopped parsley.

- Serve warm as a side dish or enjoy it on its own.

This Balsamic Roasted Cauliflower is a delicious and healthy side dish with a perfect balance of sweet and tangy flavors. Enjoy!

Dishes

Mediterranean-Style Breakfast Sweet Potato Hash

Ingredients:

- 2 large sweet potatoes, peeled and diced
- 2 tablespoons olive oil
- 1/2 red onion, finely chopped
- 1 red bell pepper, diced
- 1/2 cup cherry tomatoes, halved
- 1 cup baby spinach or kale
- 1/4 cup Kalamata olives, sliced
- 1/4 cup crumbled feta cheese
- 2 cloves garlic, minced
- 1 teaspoon dried oregano
- 1/2 teaspoon dried basil
- 1/4 teaspoon ground cumin
- Salt and black pepper, to taste
- Fresh parsley or basil, chopped (for garnish)

Instructions:

1. **Prepare the Sweet Potatoes:**
- Peel and dice the sweet potatoes into small cubes.

2. **Cook the Sweet Potatoes:**
- Heat olive oil in a large skillet over medium heat.
- Add the diced sweet potatoes and cook for 10-12 minutes, stirring occasionally, until they begin to soften and develop a golden-brown crust.

3. **Add Vegetables:**

- Add the finely chopped red onion and diced red bell pepper to the skillet.
- Cook for an additional 5-7 minutes, until the vegetables are tender and the sweet potatoes are fully cooked.

4. **Incorporate Mediterranean Ingredients:**

- Stir in the halved cherry tomatoes, sliced Kalamata olives, and minced garlic.
- Cook for another 2-3 minutes, until the tomatoes start to soften and the garlic becomes fragrant.

5. **Add Greens and Seasonings:**

- Stir in the baby spinach or kale and cook for 1-2 minutes until wilted.
- Season with dried oregano, dried basil, ground cumin, salt, and black pepper. Adjust seasoning to taste.

6. **Finish with Feta Cheese:**

- Sprinkle crumbled feta cheese over the hash and stir to combine. Let it cook for an additional minute or until the feta is slightly melted.

7. **Garnish and Serve:**

- Garnish with freshly chopped parsley or basil.
- Serve immediately, either on its own or with a side of eggs for a complete breakfast.

Enjoy your Mediterranean-style breakfast sweet potato hash!

Healthy Broccoli Egg Bake

Ingredients:

- 2 cups broccoli florets
- 1 tablespoon olive oil
- 1/2 onion, finely chopped
- 2 cloves garlic, minced
- 6 large eggs
- 1/4 cup milk or unsweetened almond milk
- 1/2 cup shredded cheddar cheese (optional for a non-dairy version)
- 1/4 cup grated Parmesan cheese
- 1/4 cup chopped fresh parsley or spinach
- 1/2 teaspoon dried oregano
- 1/4 teaspoon dried thyme
- Salt and black pepper, to taste

Instructions:

1. **Prepare the Broccoli:**

- Preheat your oven to 375°F (190°C).
- Steam or blanch the broccoli florets until tender but still vibrant, about 3-4 minutes. Drain and set aside.

2. **Sauté the Aromatics:**

- Heat olive oil in a large skillet over medium heat.
- Add the finely chopped onion and cook until softened, about 5 minutes.
- Stir in the minced garlic and cook for an additional 1 minute.

3. **Combine Ingredients:**

- In a large bowl, whisk together the eggs and milk until well combined.

- Stir in the grated Parmesan cheese, chopped parsley or spinach, dried oregano, dried thyme, salt, and black pepper.
- Gently fold in the cooked broccoli and sautéed onion and garlic mixture.

4. **Assemble the Bake:**

- Pour the egg mixture into a greased 9x9-inch baking dish or similar oven-safe dish.
- If using, sprinkle shredded cheddar cheese evenly over the top.

5. **Bake:**

- Bake in the preheated oven for 25-30 minutes, or until the eggs are set and the top is lightly golden brown.

6. **Cool and Serve:**

- Allow the egg bake to cool slightly before slicing into squares.
- Serve warm and enjoy!

This broccoli egg bake is a nutritious and delicious option for breakfast, brunch, or even a light dinner.

Bean-less Breakfast Burrito

Ingredients:

- 2 large eggs
- 1/4 cup diced bell peppers (any color)
- 1/4 cup diced onions
- 1/4 cup cooked and crumbled tilapia, turkey or chicken sausage (or ground beef for a more traditional option)
- 1/2 avocado, sliced
- 1/4 cup fresh spinach or kale
- 1 tablespoon coconut oil or olive oil
- Salt and black pepper, to taste
- Optional toppings: salsa, hot sauce, or fresh herbs

Instructions:

1. **Prepare the Ingredients:**

- Dice the bell peppers and onions.
- Slice the avocado and set aside.

2. **Cook the Vegetables and Sausage:**

- Heat coconut oil or olive oil in a skillet over medium heat.
- Add the diced onions and bell peppers to the skillet. Cook for about 5 minutes, or until the vegetables are tender.
- Add the crumbled sausage to the skillet and cook until heated through and slightly browned, about 3-4 minutes.

3. **Scramble the Eggs:**

- In a small bowl, whisk the eggs with a pinch of salt and black pepper.

- Pour the eggs into the skillet with the vegetables and sausage.

- Stir gently until the eggs are fully cooked and scrambled, about 2-3 minutes.

4. **Assemble the Burrito:**

- Lay the cooked egg mixture in the center of a large lettuce leaf (for a low-carb option) or a large gluten-free tortilla (if you prefer a traditional burrito).

- Top with fresh spinach or kale, avocado slices, and any optional toppings like salsa or hot sauce.

5. **Wrap and Serve:**

- If using a tortilla, fold in the sides and roll up the burrito tightly.

- If using a lettuce leaf, fold in the sides and roll up as you would a wrap.

Enjoy!

Parmesan Spaghetti Squash

Ingredients:

- 1 large spaghetti squash
- 2 tablespoons olive oil
- 2 cloves garlic, minced
- 1/4 cup heavy cream
- 1/2 cup grated Parmesan cheese
- 1/4 teaspoon red pepper flakes (optional)
- Salt and black pepper, to taste
- 2 tablespoons chopped fresh parsley (optional)
- Additional Parmesan cheese for garnish

Instructions:

1. **Prepare the Spaghetti Squash:**

- Preheat your oven to 400°F (200°C).
- Cut the spaghetti squash in half lengthwise and scoop out the seeds with a spoon.
- Drizzle 1 tablespoon of olive oil over the cut sides of the squash and season with salt and black pepper.
- Place the squash halves cut side down on a baking sheet lined with parchment paper.
- Roast in the oven for 30-40 minutes or until the squash is tender and easily pierced with a fork.
- Remove from the oven and let it cool slightly.

2. **Make the Sauce:**

- In a large skillet, heat the remaining 1 tablespoon of olive oil over medium heat.
- Add the minced garlic and red pepper flakes (if using) and sauté for 1 minute until fragrant.

- Stir in the heavy cream and bring it to a gentle simmer.

- Add the grated Parmesan cheese and stir until the cheese is melted and the sauce is smooth.

- Season with salt and black pepper to taste.

3. **Prepare the Spaghetti Squash:**

- Once the squash is cool enough to handle, use a fork to scrape the flesh into long strands resembling spaghetti.

4. **Combine and Serve:**

- Add the spaghetti squash strands to the skillet with the sauce and toss to coat evenly.

- Cook for an additional 2-3 minutes to warm through.

- Garnish with chopped fresh parsley and additional Parmesan cheese if desired.

- Serve immediately.

Enjoy your delicious and comforting Parmesan spaghetti squash!

Italian-Style Spaghetti Squash Shrimp Scampi

Ingredients:

- 1 large spaghetti squash
- 2 tablespoons olive oil
- 4 cloves garlic, minced
- 1/4 teaspoon red pepper flakes (optional, for heat)
- 1 pound large shrimp, peeled and deveined
- 1/4 cup dry white wine or chicken broth
- 1 tablespoon lemon juice (about 1/2 lemon)
- 1/4 cup chopped fresh parsley
- 1/4 cup grated Parmesan cheese (optional, for non-Paleo)
- Salt and black pepper, to taste
- Lemon wedges, for serving

Instructions:

1. **Prepare the Spaghetti Squash:**

- Preheat your oven to 400°F (200°C).
- Cut the spaghetti squash in half lengthwise and remove the seeds.
- Brush the cut sides with a little olive oil and season with salt and pepper.
- Place the squash cut-side down on a baking sheet lined with parchment paper.
- Roast in the preheated oven for 40-45 minutes, or until tender when pierced with a fork.

2. **Cook the Shrimp:**

- While the squash is roasting, heat olive oil in a large skillet over medium heat.

- Add the minced garlic and red pepper flakes (if using) and cook for 1 minute, until fragrant.

- Add the shrimp to the skillet and cook for 2-3 minutes per side, or until pink and cooked through. Remove the shrimp from the skillet and set aside.

3. **Make the Scampi Sauce:**

- In the same skillet, add the white wine or chicken broth and lemon juice. Bring to a simmer and cook for 2-3 minutes, allowing the liquid to reduce slightly.

- Stir in the chopped parsley and season with salt and black pepper.

4. **Prepare the Spaghetti Squash:**

- Once the squash is roasted and cool enough to handle, use a fork to scrape the flesh into spaghetti-like strands.

5. **Combine and Serve:**

- Add the cooked shrimp back into the skillet with the scampi sauce and toss to coat.

- Gently fold the spaghetti squash into the skillet and toss until everything is well combined and heated through.

- If desired, sprinkle with grated Parmesan cheese.

6. **Garnish and Enjoy:**

- Serve immediately, garnished with additional fresh parsley and lemon wedges on the side.

This Italian-style Spaghetti Squash Shrimp Scampi is a flavorful and light alternative to traditional pasta dishes, perfect for a satisfying meal!

Healthy Chicken Tacos

Ingredients:

♦ For the Chicken:

- 1 lb. boneless, skinless chicken breasts or thighs
- 1 tablespoon olive oil
- 1 teaspoon paprika
- 1 teaspoon ground cumin
- 1 teaspoon garlic powder
- 1 teaspoon onion powder
- 1/2 teaspoon chili powder
- 1/2 teaspoon dried oregano
- Salt and black pepper, to taste

♦ For the Tacos:

- 8 small corn tortillas (or whole wheat if preferred)
- 1 cup shredded lettuce or chopped romaine
- 1 cup cherry tomatoes, diced
- 1/2 cup red onion, finely chopped
- 1 avocado, sliced
- 1/4 cup fresh cilantro, chopped
- Lime wedges, for serving

♦ For the Optional Yogurt Sauce:

- 1/2 cup plain Greek yogurt
- 1 tablespoon lime juice
- 1 teaspoon honey (optional)
- 1/2 teaspoon garlic powder
- Salt and black pepper, to taste

Instructions:

1. **Prepare the Chicken:**

- In a small bowl, mix together paprika, cumin, garlic powder, onion powder, chili powder, oregano, salt, and black pepper.

- Rub the spice mixture evenly over the chicken breasts or thighs.

- Heat olive oil in a skillet over medium heat.

- Cook the chicken for 6-8 minutes per side, or until fully cooked and the internal temperature reaches 165°F (74°C).

- Remove from the skillet and let it rest for 5 minutes before slicing or shredding.

2. **Prepare the Optional Yogurt Sauce (if using):**

- In a small bowl, mix together Greek yogurt, lime juice, honey (if using), garlic powder, salt, and black pepper.

- Adjust seasoning to taste and set aside.

3. **Assemble the Tacos:**

- Warm the corn tortillas in a lightly oiled skillet or directly over a flame until pliable and slightly toasted.

- Slice or shred the cooked chicken.

- Divide the chicken among the tortillas.

- Top with shredded lettuce or chopped romaine, diced cherry tomatoes, red onion, avocado slices, and fresh cilantro.

4. **Serve:**

- Drizzle with the optional yogurt sauce if desired.

- Serve with lime wedges on the side for squeezing over the tacos.

Enjoy your healthy and clean chicken tacos!

Healthy Grilled Mediterranean-Style Hamburger

Ingredients:

♦ For the Patties:

- ♦ 1 lb ground turkey or lean ground beef
- ♦ 1/4 cup finely chopped red onion
- ♦ 1/4 cup chopped fresh parsley
- ♦ 1/4 cup crumbled feta cheese
- ♦ 1 clove garlic, minced
- ♦ 1 teaspoon dried oregano
- ♦ 1/2 teaspoon ground cumin
- ♦ Salt and black pepper, to taste

♦ For the Toppings:

- ♦ 1 cup baby spinach or mixed greens
- ♦ 1/2 cup sliced cherry tomatoes
- ♦ 1/2 cucumber, thinly sliced
- ♦ 1/4 red onion, thinly sliced
- ♦ 1/4 cup sliced Kalamata olives
- ♦ 1 tablespoon extra-virgin olive oil
- ♦ 1 tablespoon red wine vinegar

♦ For Serving:

- ♦ 4 whole wheat or gluten-free hamburger buns (optional, or lettuce wraps for a low-carb option)

Instructions:

1. Prepare the Patties:

- ♦ In a large bowl, combine ground turkey or beef with chopped red onion, parsley, crumbled feta cheese, minced garlic, dried oregano, ground cumin, salt, and black pepper.

- ♦ Mix gently until all ingredients are well combined. Avoid overmixing to keep the patties tender.

2. **Form the Patties:**

- ♦ Divide the mixture into 4 equal portions and shape each portion into a patty, about 1/2-inch thick.

3. **Preheat the Grill:**

- ♦ Preheat your grill to medium-high heat. Lightly oil the grill grates to prevent sticking.

4. **Grill the Patties:**

- ♦ Place the patties on the grill and cook for about 5-6 minutes per side, or until the internal temperature reaches 165°F (74°C) for ground turkey or 160°F (71°C) for ground beef.

5. **Prepare the Toppings:**

- ♦ In a medium bowl, toss together baby spinach or mixed greens, cherry tomatoes, cucumber, red onion, and Kalamata olives.

- ♦ Drizzle with extra-virgin olive oil and red wine vinegar. Toss to coat evenly.

6. **Assemble the Burgers:**

- ♦ If using buns, toast them lightly on the grill for 1-2 minutes.

- ♦ Top with the prepared Mediterranean salad.

- ♦ Place each patty on the bottom half of a bun or lettuce wrap.

7. **Serve:**

♦ Add the top bun or wrap and serve immediately.

Enjoy your delicious and healthy grilled Mediterranean-style hamburger!

Tuna Avocado Wrap

Ingredients:

- 2 large lettuce leaves (or whole wheat tortillas or wraps of your choice)
- 1 can (5 oz) tuna, drained
- 1 ripe avocado, peeled and pitted
- 1 tablespoon lime juice
- 2 tablespoons Greek yogurt or mayonnaise
- 1 teaspoon Dijon mustard
- Salt and pepper, to taste
- 1/4 teaspoon garlic powder
- 1/4 teaspoon onion powder
- 1/4 cup red onion, finely chopped
- 1/4 cup celery, finely chopped
- 1/4 cup cherry tomatoes, halved
- 2 cups fresh spinach or mixed greens
- 1/4 cup shredded carrots
- 1 tablespoon fresh cilantro or parsley, chopped (optional)

Instructions:

1. **Prepare the Tuna Salad:**

- In a medium bowl, mash the avocado with a fork until smooth.
- Add lime juice, Greek yogurt (or mayonnaise), and Dijon mustard to the avocado. Mix well.
- Add the drained tuna to the avocado mixture and mix until well combined.
- Season with salt, pepper, garlic powder, and onion powder. Adjust seasoning to taste.

2. **Add Vegetables:**

◆ Stir in the red onion, celery, cherry tomatoes, and cilantro or parsley (if using) into the tuna salad mixture.

3. **Assemble the Wraps:**

◆ Lay a lettuce leaf (or the whole wheat tortilla/wrap) on a clean surface.

◆ Spread half of the tuna avocado mixture in the center of the leaf.

◆ Top with 1 cup of spinach or mixed greens and 2 tablespoons of shredded carrots.

4. **Roll the Wraps:**

◆ Fold in the sides of the leaf and roll it as tightly as possible from the bottom to the top to enclose the filling.

◆ Repeat with the second leaf and remaining ingredients.

5. **Serve:**

◆ Cut each lettuce wrap in half, if desired, and serve immediately. But most importantly, enjoy your hearty and healthy tuna avocado wraps!

These wraps are perfect for a quick and nutritious lunch or dinner, packed with healthy fats and protein.

Bell Pepper Mexican Stir fry

Ingredients:

- 1 tablespoon olive oil
- 2 red bell pepper (or your favorite color pepper), chopped
- 1 cup sliced green onions, plus more for garnish
- 2 cloves garlic, minced
- 1 tablespoon chili powder
- 1 tablespoon ground cumin
- Kosher salt, to taste
- 1 pound ground beef or chicken
- 1 can (15 oz) diced tomatoes or use 3 ⅓ cups of diced tomatoes
- 1 cup canned black beans, drained and rinsed
- 1 tablespoon hot sauce
- 1/4 cup shredded Cheddar cheese for delicious garnish

Instructions:

1. Cook Vegetables:

- Heat the olive oil in a large skillet over medium-high heat.
- Add the chopped red bell pepper and sliced green onions. Cook until the vegetables are tender, about 5 minutes.

2. Add Garlic and Spices:

- Add the minced garlic to the skillet and cook until fragrant, about 1 minute.
- Stir in the chili powder and ground cumin until combined, then season with salt to taste.

3. **Cook Ground Beef:**

♦ Add the ground beef to the skillet and cook until it is no longer pink, about 5 minutes.

4. **Combine Ingredients:**

♦ Stir in the diced tomatoes and black beans until well combined.

♦ Add the hot sauce and mix thoroughly.

5. **Add Cheese:**

♦ Sprinkle the shredded Cheddar cheese over the mixture.

♦ Cover the skillet with a lid and let the cheese melt, about 1 minute.

6. **Garnish and Serve:**

♦ Garnish with additional sliced green onions before serving.

Enjoy your delicious and easy Mexican stir fry!

Asian Noodle Stir-Fry

Ingredients:

- 8 oz rice noodles (or any preferred Asian noodles)
- 2 tablespoons olive oil
- 1 boneless chicken breast or thigh, thinly sliced (optional, for added protein)
- 1 bell pepper, thinly sliced
- 1 carrot, julienned
- 1 cup snap peas
- 3 green onions, sliced
- 3 cloves garlic, minced
- 1 tablespoon ginger, minced
- 1/4 cup soy sauce (or tamari for gluten-free)
- 2 tablespoons hoisin sauce
- 1 tablespoon sesame oil
- 1 tablespoon rice vinegar
- 1 teaspoon sugar (optional, to taste)
- 1 tablespoon sesame seeds (optional, for garnish)
- Fresh cilantro or basil (optional, for garnish)

Instructions:

1. **Cook the Noodle:**

- Heat vegetable oil in a large skillet or wok over medium-high heat.
- If using chicken, add it to the skillet and cook until fully cooked and slightly browned.
- Remove and set aside.

2. **Prepare the Stir-Fry:**

- Heat vegetable oil in a large skillet or wok over medium-high heat.

- If using chicken, add it to the skillet and cook until fully cooked and slightly browned.

- Remove and set aside.

3. **Cook Vegetables:**

- In the same skillet, add a bit more oil if needed. Add garlic and ginger, cooking for about 30 seconds until fragrant.

- Add bell pepper, carrot, and snap peas.

- Stir-fry for 3-4 minutes until vegetables are tender-crisp.

4. **Combine Ingredients:**

- Return the cooked chicken (if using) to the skillet.

- Add the cooked noodles to the skillet and toss to combine with the vegetables.

5. **Garnish and Serve:**

- Remove from heat and garnish with sesame seeds and fresh cilantro or basil, if desired.

- Serve immediately.

6. **Add Sauce:**

- In a small bowl, mix together soy sauce, hoisin sauce, sesame oil, rice vinegar, and sugar (if using). Pour this sauce over the noodle and vegetable mixture.

- Toss everything together to ensure the noodles and vegetables are well-coated with the sauce.

Enjoy your flavorful and satisfying Asian noodle stir-fry!

Gluten-Free Pan-Fried Chicken Breasts

Ingredients:

- 4 boneless chicken breasts
- Olive oil (enough to coat the bottom of the frying pan)
- 1 large egg (or veganaise for an eggless version)
- 1 cup gluten-free seasoned bread crumbs
- 1/2 teaspoon garlic powder (optional, or to taste)
- Lemon wedges (for serving)
- Shaved Parmesan (optional, for garnish)
- Fresh basil (optional, for garnish)

Instructions:

1. **Prepare the Chicken:**

- Using a sharp knife, filet each chicken breast into 2 thin pieces. This will help the chicken cook faster and ensure a thinner, more flavorful result.

2. **Prepare the Coating:**

- In a bowl, scramble the egg. Alternatively, for an eggless version, use vegenaise.

- Place gluten-free seasoned bread crumbs in a separate plate or shallow dish. If desired, add garlic powder to the bread crumbs and mix well.

3. **Coat the Chicken:**

- Dip each chicken filet into the scrambled egg or veganaise, ensuring it is fully coated.

- Then, place the coated chicken filet in the gluten-free bread crumbs, pressing down lightly to ensure the crumbs adhere well to both sides.

4. **Cook the Chicken:**

♦ Heat olive oil in a frying pan over medium-high heat. The oil should be enough to thinly coat the bottom of the pan.

♦ Carefully place the breaded chicken filets into the hot oil. Cook until golden brown on both sides, approximately 3-4 minutes per side, depending on thickness.

5. **Serve:**

♦ Remove the chicken filets from the pan and place them on a paper towel-lined plate to drain excess oil.

♦ Serve with lemon wedges for a fresh burst of flavor.

♦ Optional: Garnish with shaved Parmesan and fresh sliced basil if desired.

Enjoy your delicious, gluten-free pan-fried chicken breasts!

Vegetarian Mexican Stir Fry

Ingredients:

- Olive oil
- 6 corn tortillas
- 1 green bell pepper, sliced into 1/2-inch strips
- 1 yellow bell pepper, sliced into 1/2-inch strips
- 1 orange bell pepper, sliced into 1/2-inch strips
- 1 red bell pepper, sliced into 1/2-inch strips
- 1 onion (red or white), sliced into 1/2-inch strips
- 1 can refried beans
- 3 scallions, chopped
- 1 lime, cut into wedges
- Salsa or taco sauce (optional, for garnish)

Instructions:

1. **Prepare the Vegetables:**
- Slice the bell peppers and onion into 1/2-inch strips.

2. **Cook the Vegetables:**
- Heat a tablespoon of olive oil in a cast iron or stainless steel pan over medium-high heat.
- Add the red, yellow, and orange bell peppers and the onion to the pan.
- Sauté until they are slightly blackened and charred, about 5-7 minutes.

3. **Add Refried Beans:**
- Lower the heat to medium and add the can of refried beans to the pan with the vegetables.
- Stir the mixture until all ingredients are heated through, about 1-2 minutes.

4. **Keep Warm:**

- Remove the mixture from the pan using a rubber spatula and transfer it to a bowl.

- Cover to keep it hot.

5. **Fry the Tortillas:**

- Add a little more olive oil to the pan.

- Increase the heat to high.

- Quickly pan-fry each side of the corn tortillas until they are hot and slightly crispy.

- Do this for as many tortillas as needed, adding more oil as necessary.

6. **Assemble the Dish:**

- Place two tortillas on each plate.

- Add a dollop of the bean and pepper mixture on top of the tortillas.

7. **Garnish and Serve:**

- Garnish with chopped scallions, a squeeze of lime, and a dollop of salsa or taco sauce if desired.

- Serve immediately while the tortillas are hot.

Enjoy your vibrant and flavorful Mexican stir fry!

CONCLUSION

That's a wrap on *Naturally Skinny, My Ass!* I wrote this for you with heart, humor, and hope. May it meet you right where you are and bring you practical tips, fresh inspiration, and a few loving nudges toward a more energized, healthy life. And if you take one thing with you, let it be this—healthy living should feel like freedom, not punishment. Because this isn't about perfection—it's about real-life wellness that actually fits into your day.

The best photo filter is confidence.

You can't fake the feeling of being well-fed, well-rested, and well-loved. And remember: nothing looks as good as healthy feels.

Healthy choices don't have to be complicated—just consistent, doable, and sprinkled with a little garlic and lemon, of course!

XOXO,

Denice

ENDNOTES

1. Harvard Health, "How many fruits and vegetables do we really need?" Harvard Health, September 1, 2021 https://www.health.harvard.edu/nutrition/how-many-fruits-and-vegetables-do-we-really-need.

ACKNOWLEDGEMENTS

I want to thank my brave and loving mother, who was the first to tell me that our health is our greatest wealth. As a single mom raising my brother and me on food stamps, she meant that literally!

My deep appreciation to my non-Italian husband for putting up with the pungent smells of onion, garlic, and anything fermented wafting from the kitchen for over 35 years of marriage. And a huge, teary-eyed thank you to him for constantly reminding me that not everyone was raised with the knowledge I had—and that it was my duty to get this book out there.

Special thanks to my writing coaches, editors, and encouragement engineers: Rachel Karl, Pruette Karl, and Dagmar Torres.

I also want to thank the thousands of friends I've never met, but have shared beautiful and heartfelt moments with on social media since MySpace launched in 2003. I've been sharing inspired, inexpensive ways to eat and snack healthier—and over 20 years later, I'm still friends with many of you whom I'll never hug or share a meal with in person. But you should all know that if you hadn't taken my tips, gotten healthier and leaner, and saved a few bucks in the process, I may not have been inspired enough to write this. But you did—and so I did!

I am forever grateful for your enthusiasm for a healthier, more vibrant life.

ABOUT THE AUTHOR

Denice Duff

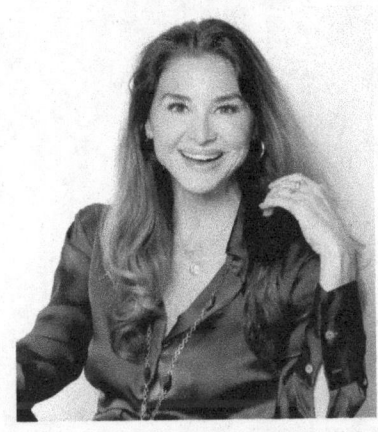

Denice Duff is an actress, director, professional photographer, and founder of the Inc. 500 skincare company IN YOUR FACE SKINCARE. She was raised by a free-spirited Italian mom in 1970s Los Angeles, growing up steeped in old-country wisdom, homegrown veggies, and holistic health long before it was trendy.

From modeling in Milan to film and soap opera sets in Hollywood, Denice has experienced the extremes of beauty culture—and now champions a more grounded, sustainable approach. Certified as a Nurse Assistant and a lifelong student of nutrition, she uses social media to share simple, affordable ways to feel good in your skin without fads or guilt.

Naturally Skinny, My Ass! is her no-hype guide to health—real, raw, and rooted in five generations of lived wisdom.

www.ingramcontent.com/pod-product-compliance
Lightning Source LLC
Chambersburg PA
CBHW010938120626
46554CB00008B/2526